Overweight Kids in a Toothpick World

How to Solve the Childhood Obesity Puzzle and Get Your *Kids in Balance*

Brenda Wollenberg

"For many years, Brenda has selflessly devoted her energies to looking for ways and means to improve the lives of others in her community. With her passion for nutrition, she has done extensive research in order to develop practical interventions to help those experiencing health issues and concerns. In her new book, Brenda translates her wide-ranging experience with nutritional counseling into a concrete program with innumerable recommendations to help those struggling with the very real challenge of childhood obesity. This well-written and thorough book will help families faced with nutritional and weight-management concerns in children to sort through the maze of information on this topic and achieve positive, life-changing outcomes."

—Stephen Genuis, MD FRCSC DABOG DABEM FAAEM
Clinical Associate Professor
Faculty of Medicine
University of Alberta

"I love your program because you have taken a very complicated issue and mapped out strategies that make healthy weight management conceivable and achievable. What these children and their families learn will stay with them for their entire lifetime. So not only does your program make an impact now, it will change their future for the better."

—Brenda Eastwood, RNCP
Registered Nutritional Consulting Practitioner
Woman's Health Specialist

"As a parent with two special needs children, maintaining good health can feel like just another of the many 'extras' that are thrown into the juggling act of parenting kids with special needs. I have often felt overwhelmed trying to implement a plan for my kids to fight physical imbalances. But what I discovered in *Kids In Balance* was an accessible program, even from the perspective of special needs. I appreciate that small changes and slow implementation is applauded and encouraged and that parents are given practical suggestions and step-by-step instructions. The principles that I learned from *KIB* give my children the advantage of a strong physically healthy platform from which to face their other challenges. I appreciate your good work!"

—Laurel A
KIB Mom

"You offer a great service to families! Our family has been a part of *KIB* for about 8 months and achieved great success! You have taught our family and daughter about making healthy choices and how to make the right balance between healthy eating and physical activity. These newly learned skills will keep her healthy for a lifetime. Thanks for a great program!"

—Naomi L
KIB Mom

"The cure to childhood obesity lies in the hands of parents. It's in the ability to say "No" to the food industry's processed food and "Yes" to natural foods that are rich in protein and good fats. *Overweight Kids in a Toothpick World* helps families address the social and emotional components to weight problems. It offers a unique and gentle way for parents to support their children achieve a healthy weight. It's well written and easy to understand presenting an easy-to-follow plan that makes sense."

—Dr. Al Sears
Founder, Center for Health and Wellness

"What you are doing is so important, and we applaud you! Our family of three has been dramatically impacted by implementing the changes that your program teaches. Before they became formalized as *KIB*, we used your principles to learn how to eat for health, change our attitudes toward life, and be an example to others of just how much a family can change with education and inspiration. Thank you! We would love to see *Kids In Balance* reach many more families with hope and success!"

—Angela K
Nutrition Client

"Jamie Oliver's Food Revolution was a good start in addressing the childhood obesity problem and Brenda Wollenberg's book takes the movement to make kids healthy further with an easy to follow plan."

—AD Rowe
Editor, *Zagasi News* (online news site)

Overweight Kids in a Toothpick World

Easy Weight Loss for
Teens and Children

OR

A Nutritionist's Step-by-Step Plan to Keep
Childhood Obesity Facts From Making Your Kid a
Childhood Obesity Statistic

Brenda Wollenberg BSW RNCP

Choices Lifestyle Publications
Langley, British Columbia

Kids in Balance Online

**For additional *Kids in Balance* information
and resources visit *KIB* online at:**

www.kidsinbalance.net

Cover and illustrations 1 and 2 by Naomi Lippett.

Library and Archives Canada Cataloguing in Publication

Wollenberg, Brenda, 1956-
     Overweight kids in a toothpick world : easy weight loss for teens and children or a nutritionist's step-by-step plan to keep childhood obesity facts from making your kid a childhood obesity statistic / Brenda Wollenberg.

Includes index.

ISBN 978-0-9866365-0-9

     1. Obesity in children--Prevention. 2. Weight loss. 3. Children--Nutrition. 4. Exercise therapy for children. I. Title.

RJ399.C6W65 2010   613.7'12   C2010-904367-7

All research and clinical material presented in this book is for informational and educational purposes only. While correct nutritional intake can provide the tools to achieve improved health and wellness, the information that follows is not intended to replace medical advice offered by health care practitioners nor intended to be used to diagnose or treat a health problem or disease.

Some of the goals and desires material taken from *The Marriage Builder* by Dr. Larry Crabb. Copyright ©1982 by Lawrence J. Crabb, Jr. Used by permission of Zondervan, www.zondervan.com.

This book is dedicated:

to Matt, Sam, Joel, Rachel and Rebekah, without whom I would not have had any supportive, humourous and amazing children on which to practise KIB-friendly recipes and lifestyle principles;

and to Mark. Every Carbohydrate Body Type needs a wonderful Protein Body Type spouse to keep things balanced. You are the best!

Acknowledgments

Thanks to Anne Marie for her perspective and passion in the initial stages of *Kids in Balance*. Coming up with an effective, family friendly plan to tackle childhood obesity would have been a lot less fun and contained fewer tasty recipes if you hadn't decided to pick up the phone and give me a call.

Thanks to Cheryl and Laurel, my exceedingly kind but lovingly honest editing sister and friend—the long sentences are for you.

Thanks Nae for lots of things: for being in this for the long haul, for getting what I'm about and for capturing the essence of *KIB* in such a creative and colorful way.

Thanks as well to Christy. What can I say my friend? You have brought fresh insight to this project, and an eye for clarity, detail and cohesion that is exceedingly appreciated. Next time you ask, "Do you want brilliant?" I might groan, but I'd probably take you up on it again.

And finally, thanks to my nutrition clients and *KIB* families. You are the inspiration for this book—working with you brings smiles to my day!

Note that the names in many of the testimonials have been changed to respect confidentiality.

Table of Contents

About This Book

Most parents of a child carrying excess weight recognize that an unhealthy or overabundant diet and insufficient physical activity contribute to obesity. If you are one of many parents, however, who has tried unsuccessfully to use that knowledge to help your child, you are not alone.

- ❏ Many parents feel they have failed in their ability to move their child to a state of health and wellness with regard to weight.
- ❏ Many parents feel they have been misjudged or at the least, unsupported, in their attempts to stem their child's weight gain.
- ❏ Many parents feel confused over which nutritional and weight loss information to implement with their child.
- ❏ Many parents feel any attempts they have made to assist their child shed excess weight have worked minimally or, in fact, have led to increased weight gain.
- ❏ Many parents do not understand why some of their children are in a healthy weight range and yet one or more carry excess weight.
- ❏ Many parents feel they are missing vital pieces of information that seem to be contributing factors to their child's excess weight.

If you are experiencing any of those thoughts or emotions, the *Kids in Balance* (*KIB*) program described in this book can help.

Parents researching the causes and solutions for childhood obesity have discovered that information on this topic is vast, confusing and often contradictory. Though *Kids in Balance* is based on the most natural, sound and effective parts of that information, in order to keep the program as understandable and attainable as possible, the content in this book has been kept simple. In fact, kept B-A-L-A-N-C-E simple.

The wide range of childhood obesity information has been distilled to seven primary problems and seven essential solutions that can easily be remembered using the BALANCE acronym:

B - **B**ody type
A - **A**ttitude
L - **L**aughter and play
A - **A**ctivity
N - a good **N**ight's sleep
C - **C**lean water
E - **E**at for health

Not only does this book explain the BALANCE principles in detail, it also offers a simple to follow, 3-Phase Program for parents and guardians who want to help their children "**Find their BALANCE**," "**Build their BALANCE**" and "**Keep their BALANCE**" for life.

Kids in Balance 3-Phase Program	
Phase 1 **Find Your BALANCE** *INTENSITY*	❏ Duration: One week of preparation and three weeks of Phase 1. ❏ Primary preparation tasks are reading, learning and understanding. ❏ Primary **Find Your BALANCE** tasks are attitude and food adjustment. ❏ First week of phase is gradual dietary and lifestyle change. ❏ Second and third week are a gentle dietary cleanse. ❏ *Day-at-a-Glance Guidelines* walk you through each step of the *Kids in Balance* journey.
Phase 2 **Build Your BALANCE** *PERSEVERENCE*	❏ Duration: Depending upon amount of excess weight your child is carrying, **Build Your BALANCE** phase can last 1-12 months or more. ❏ Primary task is consistently healthy dietary choices, per **Body** type, with room for a modest amount of exceptions. ❏ Secondary task is **Activity**—in various forms—as a lifestyle. ❏ **Attitude, Laughter** and play, **Clean** water and a good **Night's** sleep are also important **Build Your BALANCE** components.
Phase 3 **Keep Your BALANCE** *FREEDOM*	❏ Duration: **Keep Your BALANCE** lasts forever. ❏ Primary task is maintenance but, in general, the *KIB* approach has now become easy second nature. ❏ The array of *KIB* tools ensures weight is maintained in an appropriate range and that increased wellness is achieved. ❏ Health truly is in your home.

If you or your child want to do further research or explore more of the underpinnings of the program, you are welcome to check out the DIGGING DEEPER sidebars throughout the book. For just the nuts and bolts of the *KIB* approach, stick to the basics, and leave the sidebars for later.

Childhood obesity is a widespread and increasing problem. Despite the challenging degree and rate of growth of the obesity issue, however, every child deserves a chance at wellness. As a parent, you have both the privilege and the responsibility of helping your child find their way through unhelpful societal norms on the journey to better health.

Real food. Real bodies. Real health. If those sound like principles you and your child can embrace then read on! Check out the *Kids in Balance* game plan and discover what other families are saying about their positive and life-changing *KIB* results. Then take the simple steps toward lifestyle change that will allow your child to shed excess weight and arrive at and maintain a state of healthy balance and wellness.

Chapter 1

Kids in Balance Foundations

A sailor without a destination cannot hope for a favorable wind.

Leon Tec M.D.

The *Kids in Balance* approach to childhood obesity rests on four cornerstone beliefs: obesity is a widespread and increasing problem; every child deserves a chance at wellness; parents have both the responsibility and privilege of care for their children; and societal norms are not necessarily helpful.

Obesity—Widespread and Increasing

Approximately 30% of North American children are overweight and more than 10% are obese. Those numbers are climbing. Obesity can put an individual at risk for many health challenges including Type II diabetes, high blood pressure, high cholesterol, cancer and cardiovascular disease. Understanding the factors that contribute to obesity means more effectively putting a game plan in place to counteract those factors and more easily helping your child transition to an appropriate weight and optimal health.

There is a great deal of research on the various factors contributing to the past three decades' steady rise in childhood obesity rates. These health statistics lead to the first cornerstone of *KIB*'s approach to health and wellness—the belief that childhood obesity is a far-reaching and growing problem that needs to be addressed now.

In 2004, the World Health Organization commissioned the International Obesity Task Force (IOTF) to research and document the key factors at play in rising obesity rates. The list is extensive. Here, in an excerpt from **"Obesity in children and young people: A crisis in public health,"** (published in the journal *Obesity Reviews*, May 2004) are their key conclusions as to problematic trends contributing to the issue:

"Increase in use of motorized transport, e.g. to school.
Fall in opportunities for recreational physical activity.
Increased sedentary recreation.
Multiple TV channels around the clock.
Greater quantities and variety of energy dense foods available.
Rising levels of promotion and marketing of energy-dense foods.
More frequent and widespread food purchasing opportunities.
More use of restaurants and fast food stores.
Larger portions of food offering better "value" for money.
Increased frequency of eating occasions.
Rising use of soft drinks to replace water, e.g. in schools.

Stronger policies are needed to:

Provide clear and consistent consumer information, e.g. on food labels;
Encourage food companies to provide lower energy, more nutritious foods marketed for children;
Develop criteria for advertising that promotes healthier eating;
Improve maternal nutrition and encourage breast-feeding of infants;
Design secure play facilities and safe local neighbourhoods;
Encourage schools to enact coherent food, nutrition and physical activity policies;
Encourage medical and health professionals to participate in the development of public health programmes."

The more one researches the issues contributing to childhood obesity, the clearer it becomes that a multi-pronged approach will be needed to return our children to health. Fortunately, with *Kids in Balance*, parents have a program that addresses the primary contributing factors to childhood obesity and presents that comprehensive plan in a simple and effective manner.

DIGGING DEEPER
Childhood Obesity

I could produce a whole book on "digging deeper" into the issues of childhood obesity. Most parents of a child carrying excess weight, however, already know childhood obesity is an issue and have some understanding of the many contributing factors—including the main challenges, overeating of unhealthy foodstuffs and insufficient activity—to the increasing epidemic. For this reason, the *Kids in Balance* program is heavily weighted on the side of presenting practical solutions to this challenge. For parents still in research mode, however, or for those who simply like to stay abreast of the issue, here are places to go for research information; I may not agree with all of the information on these sites but they are good places to start:

Find information on childhood obesity for both parents and healthcare providers at www.aap.org/obesity/index.html, the website for the America Academy of Pediatrics. There is a childhood obesity-focused journal issue of The Princeton-Brookings Future of Children at www.futureofchildren.princeton.edu/summaries/obesity.asp. And if your interest is in helping fight obesity in the public school system, check out www.futureofchildren.princeton.edu/briefs/briefs/FOC policy brief spr 06.pdf where Future of Children also provides a policy brief on this topic.

A Chance at Wellness

Almost without exception (i.e. rare medical conditions, extreme poverty), children have the potential to be at a healthy weight. This principle—though short and simple in nature—has wide-reaching ripple effects. If children have the potential to be at a healthy weight, the myth of "once an obese child, always an obese child," is quickly debunked. Being obese no longer has to be the norm, and children no longer need to be bound by genetics or circumstance.

In addition, *KIB*'s cornerstone belief that all children deserve a chance at wellness has a sub point. Not only do children deserve and have potential to be at a healthy weight, *KIB* believes it is possible to **safely** transition a child—both physically and emotionally—to that balanced state. With the proper attitude and information, there is enormous potential for a child to improve self-esteem and find body balance and well being. It starts by acknowledging your child's excess weight and then together with her, developing a plan to deal with that health challenge.

Believing every child should have the opportunity for good health is one thing. Coming up with a game plan that actually provides the attainable stepping stones to move a child from obesity to an appropriate weight range is another!

A good starting place is grasping the seven primary problems I see contributing to excess weight and understanding the steps needed to address each of those factors. That knowledge goes a long way to putting all children on a level playing field and to providing the opportunity for everyone to receive the health benefits that go along with reaching and maintaining a healthy weight.

Parental Responsibility and Privilege

KIB's philosophy is that the main responsibility for an overweight child's weight loss belongs with the parents or primary caregivers. I suspect that since you are reading this book, you most likely feel that way too. While there are many factors that influence weight—genetics, lifestyle and emotions to name a few—it is important for parents to do everything within their ability to move a child toward, and maintain her in, her healthiest state. Parents are privileged because they are usually the most positive influence and strongest guiding force in a child's life. Generally they are ideally positioned to guide a child through lifestyle transition.

When you begin the *KIB* program, I suggest partnering in the responsibilities that lie ahead and appropriately dividing up tasks. As a parent, you are authorized with the primary care for your child's health. You have the maturity and skill set to sort through information and wisely set a course of action as to diet and lifestyle. Just as with homework and chore expectations, it is fitting to expect compliance with what you and your child agree to in terms

---

DIGGING DEEPER
Parenting

One of my absolute favourite resources with regard to parents' ability to bring positive change and health to their children's body, mind and spirit, is Gordon Neufeld and Gabor Maté's *Hold on to Your Kids*. Written by a clinical psychologist and a physician, in a clear, insightful and imminently practical manner, the tools and suggestions made in *Hold on to Your Kids* will go a long way toward ensuring a wise grasp on the topic of parent/child relationships. The book presents a strong foundation for all types of health—body, mind and spirit.

of food intake and daily routines such as bedtimes and activity levels. Helping your family reach optimal wellness is not your job alone, however. Share the responsibility with your child, and be sure to make use of the support offered by *KIB* in this book and at www.kidsinbalance.net.

Once you and your child understand your job descriptions (see Figure 1), there is better awareness of how you will work together to succeed at the *Kids in Balance* program.

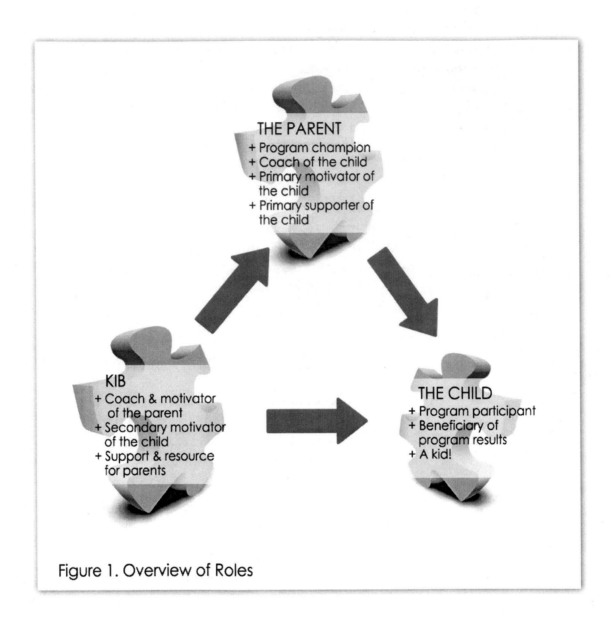

THE PARENT
+ Program champion
+ Coach of the child
+ Primary motivator of the child
+ Primary supporter of the child

KIB
+ Coach & motivator of the parent
+ Secondary motivator of the child
+ Support & resource for parents

THE CHILD
+ Program participant
+ Beneficiary of program results
+ A kid!

Figure 1. Overview of Roles

Societal Norms

Today's commonly accepted lifestyle and cultural practices do not necessarily support reaching or maintaining a healthy weight. We currently live in an era of fast rather than slowly and nutritionally prepared food; rapidly increasing sugar intake; role models that include underweight models and bulimic celebrities; and a poor ratio of physical activity to screen time—the amount of time spent watching television, on the computer, texting or playing video games.

The *KIB* approach is designed to counteract those unhealthy realities with a back to basics lifestyle change and realistic health goals. And the approach is geared for a family setting. Why? Because ultimately I believe, and statistics seem to confirm, that changes in simple household routines can be key to whether a child is overweight or not,[1,2] and that dietary and lifestyle change is most effective when both parents and children are involved in the process.[3]

The last of the four cornerstones in *KIB*'s approach to wellness is the recognition that, in many ways, families seeking to simply and naturally improve the health of their children are working in direct opposition to much of today's culture. Currently, almost all that our children see, hear and are exposed to, directs them toward an increased intake of foods that produce decreased wellness; the acquisition of technological gear that takes time from physical activity; and the promotion of a busy life of doing and having everything—all factors that contribute to ill health and excess weight. At the same time, through advertising, the entertainment industry and even peer relationships, children receive the mixed message of the need to attain a "toothpick" body shape.

Additionally, the careful thought, time and energy required to really attend to a family—body, mind and spirit—is near the bottom of most people's priority lists. A family valuing a slower, simpler and more back to basics lifestyle is like a salmon swimming upstream: life will be challenging, have rough patches and produce good results, but almost everyone else will be going in the opposite direction!

It is true there are encouraging signs on the horizon—the removal of pop machines from schools, more accurate nutritional labels on packaged foods, the arrival of vegetables at fast food restaurants, an increased appearance of realistic body shapes in the media—but in general, making significant lifestyle change that will actually position you and your family for real health, is going to move you away from many of the norms of most other families. Even something as simple as putting forward the request that your child not be rewarded with penny candy or suckers at school, club or youth group could be a challenge.

Fortunately, while families following a quality, natural approach to health and wellness may be in the minority, their numbers are definitely on the increase, and the priorities of more and more parents are changing. As they then teach their children to recognize and avoid the foods, products and activities that undermine health—and encourage them to have a hearty skepticism of the reality and healthfulness of images portrayed around them—we will hopefully see that the majority of the salmon are going in the most life-producing, even if still challenging, direction!

Who Does Well on the *KIB* Program?

What I have discovered over the past number of years is that while virtually everyone who follows the *Kids in Balance* program garners improved health and wellness, *KIB* works optimally in certain family settings and with certain types of children.

First, by virtue of the fact you are reading this book, it is very likely that yours is a family that would do well on the *KIB* program. Recognizing your child needs help in the area of weight management, taking time to evaluate the different ways of tackling childhood obesity and being willing to explore a program of lifestyle change usually indicates:

❑ You are ready to make change and are prepared to do the work that change requires.

❑ You understand that excess weight is not gathered in a short period of time and that, therefore, reaching a healthy balanced state will require longer-term effort.

❑ You are prepared to take responsibility for your family's health and realize that the food you are putting in your mouths is growing your bodies.

❑ You realize there are a number of factors contributing to your child's excess weight and want more than a one-shot or magic bullet approach.

As the parent, you will set the tone and provide the guidelines for lifestyle change, but your child has a role to play as well. Accordingly, I have found that the children who have the most resounding success on the *KIB* program:

❑ Are between the ages of 5-18.

❑ Are fairly willing to make some changes in diet and lifestyle.

❑ Feel a need for change because of health challenges or other difficulties (i.e. emotional, relational) they are experiencing because of the excess weight.

Finally, for both parents and children, those that do well with the *Kids in Balance* approach understand that while there will be effort involved in following the *KIB* program, the end results will be well worth it!

Benefits of the *KIB* Program

Though the *KIB* program is simple and effective, it can have its challenging moments. Therefore, before embarking on a journey that will require some degree of discipline and lifestyle adjustment, it is important to understand and be encouraged by the benefits of the program.

Attainable Game Plan—*KIB* believes that the parent or primary caregiver is the best person to guide a child through lifestyle transition, and that lifestyle change is most effective when undertaken by the whole family. It is also common knowledge, however, that everyone can use a little help sometimes. The *KIB* program is a coaching plan designed to give parents the step-by-step information needed to safely transition their child from an excess weight to a healthy, balanced state. *KIB* resources are designed to turn the tough job of raising a healthy family into a manageable and attainable reality.

Proper Equipment—Completing a task well requires the right tools. In order to facilitate safe, appropriate and long lasting weight loss and maintenance, your family will need equipment that increases knowledge (i.e. factors that contribute to unhealthy weight gain), equipment that encourages enthusiasm (i.e. ideas to help your child stay motivated through lifestyle change), as well as equipment to assist you and your child through each step of the *Kids in Balance* 3-Phase Program. With *KIB*'s customized tool bag of menu plans, recipes, shopping tips, activity suggestions and more, you will have everything you need to best work with your child.

Quality Information—The *Kids in Balance* approach is based on years of experience in working with families and individuals dealing with eating/weight issues. Besides nutritional and fitness instructor training and my years in private practise as a Registered Nutritional Consulting Practitioner, I have almost a decade of experience in the field of social work and have understanding as to the ways that emotions, attitude and activity affect weight and health. By combining educational skills and personal strengths I have developed a program that recognizes the many issues that contribute to childhood obesity and provides a concrete strategy to direct your family to a place of health and balance.

Wholesome Food—The *KIB* program is simply and flavourfully based on eating appropriate amounts and types of whole, natural and quality foods. Factors such as body type and *KIB* phase— terms that will shortly be defined—guide the serving size and type of proteins, carbohydrates and fats your child will eat. And regardless of body type or program phase, a wide range of easily attainable real food is included. Once the ingredients in *KIB*'s *Healthy Foods Lists* are combined in delicious *KIB* Recipes or substituted into your own family favourites, you will find eating the *Kids in Balance* way becomes easy and tasty second nature.

Affordable Cost—The *KIB* program is explained in a cost effective book and makes use of real food, purchased from regular sources: grocery stores, produce shops and farmers' markets. Following the *KIB* program, especially if you make use of the information in *KIB on a Budget* (p. 199), should be an attainable choice for most families.

Obesity is a widespread and increasing problem; every child deserves a chance at wellness; parents have both the responsibility and privilege of care for their children; and societal norms are not necessarily helpful. If these four cornerstone beliefs do not particularly resonate with you, then you can probably save yourself a lot of time by putting down this book and trying to deal with your child's excess weight in another manner. If, however, the beliefs make sense to you, and you are looking for a simple step-by-step family wellness plan built on those cornerstones, then you are in the right place.

KIB Stories for Life

After three months of diligent Build Your BALANCE phase effort, Rebekah feels like a brand new person and really enjoys the sensation of being an "average-weight" child.

Now, she can focus more on the rest of her life. She joined synchronized swimming and makes daily efforts toward being active and balancing food intake. She started taking healthy risks and has blossomed quickly in her new confidence. Most of all, she continues in her new lifestyle, knowing it is the best way to hold on to her success. She never forgets how hard she worked for it!

Lynette

Chapter 2

Seven Big Problems – Seven BALANCE Solutions

Focus 90% of your time on solutions and only 10% of your time on problems.

Anthony J. D'Angelo
Educational Entrepreneur

While governments are working on implementing stronger obesity prevention policies, especially around food marketing and labeling, my goal is to help address childhood obesity issues that are within a parent and child's ability to change. In my evaluation of the research and my years of working with parents and children, I have found there are seven primary factors contributing to excess weight in most obese and overweight children.

Seven Problems Contributing to Childhood Obesity

One Size Fits All Philosophy—Every body is different—metabolism, inherent genetic strengths and weakness, nutritional requirements, hormonal challenges—and recommending the same dietary and lifestyle changes for everyone simply does not work. When a non-individualized plan is implemented there are rarely positive and long lasting wellness effects. The resulting discouragement and frustration can actually lead to increased weight and additional health issues.

A lack of recognition of, and appreciation for, our vast differences in physical and emotional make-up can also contribute to the belief that one particular size is the ideal. *KIB* counters society's love affair with a "toothpick" body shape, the book title's reference to a world that idolizes an unnatural, unrealistic-to-maintain and overly slender physical appearance. While there are certainly naturally very slim and healthy people, *Kids in Balance* recognizes and, in fact, celebrates, the value of different body types, including the denser, rounder and often-heavier body type—the Protein Body Type—described later in the book. As you and your child grow in your understanding of body types and in how to bring your child, whatever his body type, to a place of increased health, wellness and appropriate body size, I hope to debunk the discouraging and often health-destroying belief of toothpick body as ideal. By setting realistic body shape goals, eating appropriate types and amounts of real food, and avoiding the yo-yo dieting that yearnings for a too-thin body can often produce, you should find your child settling into a healthier weight range and growing in the sense of feeling comfortable in his own skin.

Belief Systems—In weight maintenance—as well as in every other element of body, mind and spirit wellness—attitudes and beliefs greatly influence health. Negative self-image, poor self-esteem, little sense of worthiness, minimal expectation of success and poorly designed motivators all impact one's ability to reach and maintain a healthy weight.

Stress—When adrenal glands are stressed in particular ways they produce hormones that challenge the body's ability to shed stored fat. Additionally, low protein and fatty acid intake, and decreased serotonin levels in the brain can contribute to the emotional stress of depression that in turn can contribute to cravings for sweets and starchy foods. If underlying stress factors are not dealt with, long-term healthy weight maintenance is unlikely.

Emotional and environmental stressors also impact liver function. The liver has many functions including processing hormones, eliminating toxins, cleaning the blood, metabolizing proteins and carbohydrates into energy, and manufacturing bile to help break down fats. It is important to keep the liver functioning well so the many jobs it does—including the jobs that contribute to healthy weight maintenance—can be tackled appropriately.

Lack of Exercise—Exercise plays a variety of roles in combating excess weight, including assistance with stress relief and hormone regulation. Exercise also burns calories and builds muscle, both of which are required for maintaining a healthy weight. Exercise of all types—functional and active—needs to be part of a healthy lifestyle.

Lack of Sleep—Without adequate sleep, the body shows signs of increased stress, a contributing factor to weight gain. In addition, the hormone regulation that the body utilizes to both reduce and increase hunger and carbohydrate cravings requires adequate amounts of sleep to function properly.

Insufficient Water—Water intake is essential for life. Insufficient intake drastically impacts the body's ability to maintain healthy organ function, digestion and weight. Substituting pop, coffee, juice and most teas for water compounds the problem.

Food Choices—Though there are many poor food decisions that contribute to excess weight, one of the primary impacts on obesity is the North American—and internationally spreading—dietary emphasis on "toothpick" fuel. Can you imagine if you and your child were on an overnight hike and tried to build a campfire using only toothpicks? The flame may burn bright for a moment but inevitably would be extinguished without lasting effect. Foodstuffs such as refined grains and sugars that are broken down rapidly by the body; provide little nutritional benefit; spike blood sugar levels; and, among other things, set a child up for increased rates of hunger, overeating and increased excess weight, are the core of this book title's second meaning for "toothpick" world.

Not only does the *KIB* program work to put the toothpick body shape in its proper not-a-reality place, *Kids in Balance* also teaches you and your child how to minimize the intake of toothpick foods and instead, to eat a fuel mix of whole foods that nourish, satisfy and create a long-lasting sense of what *KIB* calls Comfortable Fullness.

Amount of vegetable and fruit intake also impacts your child's ability to reach and maintain a healthy weight. Among other effects, insufficient intake of vegetables and other foods high in phytochemicals—healthful plant compounds—impacts the body's ability to regulate blood vessel growth. According to current research—much of which is being done through the Angiogenesis Foundation (www.angio.org/index.php)—extensive angiogenesis (too many blood vessels), supplies an abundance of nutrients that can fuel a variety of diseases, including obesity.[1,2] See the Angiogenesis Foundation website for a list of *Antiangiogenic Foods that Fight Cancer and Obesity*, or simply eat the *KIB* way. Many of the vegetables, fruits and oils listed at the Foundation's site are *Kids in Balance* dietary recommendations, including one of my favourites, dark chocolate. That means the healthful properties of these antiangiogenesis foods, including their ability to help regulate blood vessel growth and, in turn, help decrease body fat, are a natural part of the *KIB* program.

Additional food choice issues can also contribute to weight gain. These factors include over-eating, food sensitivities and excess sugar and grain consumption, particularly for body types that require a higher proportion of fat and protein-rich foods in their diet to reach satiety.

Ultimately, each child struggling with excess weight will have a very personalized combination of reasons for their inability to shed that excess weight, but I have found that most of these seven primary factors—and usually all—will need to be properly addressed before a balanced healthy weight can be achieved and maintained. The BALANCE acronym of the *Kids in Balance* program name is designed to address each of those seven factors—**B**ody type, **A**ttitude, **L**aughter and play, **A**ctivity, a good **N**ight's sleep, **C**lean water and **E**at for health.

As much as it can feel somewhat daunting to have so many problems influencing your child's weight, the encouragement is that you have control over most of those seven factors. *You* help set attitude and instruct about the ability to make good choices. *You* determine the serious or playful tone in your household and both model and teach ways to deal with stress. *You* are an example of and encourager in how to stay physically fit. *You* establish and ensure compliance with bedtimes. *You* provide the beverages of choice in your household and influence how much water is consumed. *You* are most likely the primary grocery shopper and food preparer in your home. And while you cannot determine which body typing factors are inherited and expressed in your child, *you* can help your child understand his body type and learn to eat the fuel mix that optimizes health.

There is no way around it: the person that is largely responsible for the health and well being of your child is you, his parent or primary caregiver. And while, at the end of the day, it is your responsibility to do the research; sort through the information; determine what seems best for your child; and then implement a plan of action that helps your child reach his goals, with the *Kids in Balance* 3-Phase Program and support materials, you do not have to handle those tasks alone.

KIB Stories for Life

It's been almost 5 years since Beth began this journey, and while she has normal teenage struggles with food choices and fitting exercise into an active social life, she is still living the lifestyle and is still experiencing changes. One thing is for sure; she is in charge of her body and there's no going back.

Rhonda

KIB's 3-Phases to Success

Because *KIB* addresses a range of problems contributing to childhood obesity, it covers a lot of material. As well, supporting families in a lifestyle rather than a one-shot approach to health, takes time. Therefore, like any extended and multifaceted journey, *KIB* is best broken down into stages—in this case, **Find Your BALANCE**, **Build Your BALANCE** and **Keep Your BALANCE** phases.

Phase 1—Find Your BALANCE—KIB's first phase is prefaced by one week of preparation and includes three weeks of gradual lifestyle modification. Through helpful information in the **Find Your BALANCE** chapter and in the *Day-at-a-Glance Guidelines* (p. 223), during the preparation week, both you and your child will be growing in your understanding of healthy living and in awareness of food's impact on mood, energy and weight. There will also be short, simple homework assignments that help your family get firmly started on the healthy living journey. During the first week of **Find Your BALANCE**, the *Day-at-a-Glance Guidelines* begin to incorporate gradual dietary change that will slowly transition your child from refined sugar and grain intake. The steps prepare your child for the last two weeks of **Find Your BALANCE** and their increased level of lifestyle change. This phase is of short duration but is fairly **intense** both in changes from the Standard North American Diet and in need for more precise adherence to *KIB* guidelines.

Phase 2—Build Your BALANCE—This phase lasts as long as it takes your child to move into a healthy weight range. That duration depends upon a number of factors including the amount of excess weight your child is carrying; body type; adherence to proper food intake ratios; and amount and intensity of activity. In addition, the attention you pay to factors beyond food intake and activity (i.e. attitude, laughter and play, water intake, sleep), and the fact that everyone is a unique individual means your child's journey to wellness will not necessarily follow the same timeline as that of another child. While vigilance with regard to the seven *KIB* components continues to be extremely important, there is some relaxation in the inclusion of all *KIB* Healthy Living Pyramid food groups (see p. 64), including minimal amounts of Sometimes Foods—foods that may not be optimal fuel for your child but that he may, on occasion, choose to enjoy. This phase is of longer duration and would be characterized by the word **perseverance**.

Phase 3—Keep Your BALANCE—The final phase of the *Kids in Balance* program lasts for as long as you, the parent, are responsible for the health of your child. This phase is marked by a sense of moderation and liberty, as healthy behaviour patterns become more a natural lifestyle. By this point in the program, there is a great deal of understanding about your child's unique body traits and the various methods needed to keep moving your child toward optimal health. There is also an acceptance of the natural rhythms of life and the need to balance seasons of slight excess (i.e. holidays, celebrations) with periods of increased self-discipline (i.e. adding in a couple of **Find Your BALANCE** days upon return from a week at an all-inclusive resort). This phase is best described as a **freedom** phase and will hopefully not only be part of your child's life for as long as he resides at home but will be carried with him as a health and wellness inheritance for life.

KIB's 3-Phase Program looks at the primary problems contributing to childhood obesity and clearly articulates how to incorporate the BALANCE solutions into an easy to follow game plan. All you have to do is read through the next few chapters to find out a little more about each BALANCE factor and then, along with your child, start taking the small steps outlined for each phase.

Seven Solutions for Childhood Obesity

B-A-L-A-N-C-E

When helping a child struggling with excess weight, it is not enough to merely pinpoint the problems contributing to childhood obesity. *Kids in Balance,* therefore, goes beyond simple identification and links each of the seven problems with seven solutions.

Body Type

Every body is different and needs its own ratio of macronutrients—proteins, carbohydrates and fats. Ancestry and genetics help determine body type and give clues as to correct fuel mix.

Attitude

Thinking positively, feeling a need for change and having a good attitude about the adjustments needed to become healthy are important keys to reaching goals.

Laughter & Play

Humour is not merely something to set you and your child chuckling! It can lower blood pressure, reduce stress, increase muscle flexibility and boost immune function. And controlling stress also helps reduce excess weight. Want to hear a good joke?

Activity

Physical exercise generally improves sleep and can help make one cheerier, stronger and more flexible. Need additional reasons to join a soccer team or walk rather than catch a ride to school? Activity helps burn fat and can make the brain work better too. As Nike so aptly advocates, "Just do it!"

A Good Night's Sleep

Skimping on sleep can mean decreased brain functioning, less energy and excess weight. Pre-teens need about 10 hours of sleep per night, and adolescents about 9.5 hours.

Clean Water

Water is our body's transportation method for getting nutrients to cells and carrying waste away from cells. It lubricates our joints, keeps us from overheating and helps our food digest. Clean water is also one of the best natural protections against a variety of infectious diseases.

Eat for Health

Eat real food, eat it as close as possible to its natural form and do not become a food fanatic. Then follow suggestions made in **Food Fundamentals** (p. 59) and you are on your way to growing a trim, healthy body.

Chapter 3

B - BODY TYPE

Eating for one's individual metabolism is a time-tested truth . . . celebrate your uniqueness, even if it is with foods shunned by conventional paradigms.

Robert. J. Rowen, M.D.

Now that you have a beginning understanding of the *Kids in Balance* approach—**B**ody type, **A**ttitude, **L**aughter and play, **A**ctivity, a good **N**ight's sleep, **C**lean water and **E**at for health—it is time to explore in greater detail each of the potential contributing factors to your child's excess weight.

Why I am a Huge Fan of Body Typing
(or how I got my svelte and happy husband back)

For the first 10 years of my own optimal health journey, I studied, wrote, taught and dragged my mostly willing family down the road of less processed foods, more fresh fruits and vegetables, and less sugar and white flour. We all felt a lot better, had more energy, slept more soundly and were at reasonably healthy weights. Then, based on some of the research I was doing, I decided to fine-tune things a bit and have everyone increase their already great level of health (or so I thought). For two years, therefore, I moved us to a vegetarian diet. I enjoyed ensuring our family was getting the proper level of important nutrients through legumes, nuts and seeds, hearty whole grains, a small amount of healthy unsaturated fat and lots of fruits and vegetables; found the international-style recipes I was using to be tasty and well-balanced; and loved all the salads and fruit smoothies. Frankly, I felt amazing.

My head was clearer than ever; my organizational capabilities and the ability to accomplish my extensive daily to-do list soared; and my energy was matched only by my easy ability to stay at a toned, slim body shape. It was clear that the Wollenberg family had found the perfect dietary plan, and I shifted my nutritional recommendations, both written and spoken, to that effect.

Unfortunately not everyone in my family was experiencing the same wonderful health benefits I had seen. While most of our kids were doing all right on the dietary plan, our oldest had been noted to have some attention and learning challenges at school, and the suggestion had been made that he be put on medication. And my husband, Mark, was not doing well at all. A 6'2" ex-high school and college football, basketball and volleyball player, Mark weighed 240 pounds at his appropriate weight; I used to joke that he had thighs the size of my waist. Mark is of German descent and had grown up eating meat eighteen times a day. Well, perhaps that is a bit of an exaggeration—let's just say he had grown up eating a lot of family farm-raised meat!

By the time we had wrapped up year two of our move to vegetarianism, Mark had put on 20 pounds, most of it in that gut-hanging-over-the-belt abdominal region. That, however, was the least of his problems. He was more fatigued, less focused, always hungry, had swapped channel surfing for our usual after supper walk or game of tennis, and was cranky. Really cranky.

Ever in investigative mode, one day I came across material on the concept of body typing—the underpinnings for the belief that a one-size-fits-all diet may not actually be a sound idea. The author presented data showing the varied historical diets of indigenous people groups from around the world and then presented statistics showing health decline once those groups began moving to a diet that seriously shifted the weighting of the various components of their original diets. I had already seen the research on the negative health shift of people moving to a diet high in refined sugars and processed foods. I also easily made sense of the information that showed poor health results when moving a vegetarian people group to a high dietary intake of meat and fat. What absolutely astonished me, however, was seeing the health decline of people with a strongly inherited need for animal protein and higher fat intake in their diet, when they moved to a low-fat, vegetarian diet. The negative changes of moving to what I had considered to be the ultimate in a healthy diet were an exact description of what I had been ignoring in my own household for almost two years.

In the midst of my research, I called Mark over to take a simple survey contained in the book I was reading and then totaled his scores. In the fifteen years since that day, having administered that survey, or ones like it, to hundreds of clients and attendees at my nutrition seminars, I have never had anyone score as high in the column showing need for dietary animal protein as Mark did that day. Our son experiencing attention challenges in school also showed need for a higher animal protein and fat intake. As Mark handed his survey back to me, I shook my head slowly, still trying to process all the new information but shortly thereafter announced it made sense to look into buying some non-medicated, grass fed beef. I think my exact words were: "Well, I guess we need to go buy you a cow." Rarely had I seen such rejoicing in our household, at least over something as simple as what to add to the grocery list.

As one who tries not to hold on to "truths" that simply do not play out in real life, when my philosophy on what constituted proper nutrition shifted, so too did my day-to-day practices:

- For my family members that showed a need for increased animal protein and fat intake, I began to incorporate, on a regular basis, small amounts of healthily raised beef, bison, poultry, lamb, fattier fish and eggs into their diet, and reduced their grain intake.
- Body type surveys became part of the standard intake form package for my nutritional consulting practise.
- I stopped moving all my clients to a vegetarian diet and only suggested a diet of that type to clients that had a similar body type to mine (when I did the survey I scored very high in the Carbohydrate Body Type category and thus my wonderful results on a vegetarian diet).
- I became a firm believer in the one-size-does-not-fit-all dietary plan and worked to ensure my clients knew that if they truly wanted to reach a healthy weight and achieve optimal health, each of them was going to need to pay attention to his or her body and learn to work with its unique needs.

And how, you might be wondering, did Mark do when we added back in appropriate proportions of animal protein and fat to his diet each day? I had a cheerier and comfortably full husband almost immediately; his energy began to return to normal pre-vegetarian diet levels within a week or two; procrastination and apathy (i.e. toward things like extra household projects) began to diminish; and within two months, he had dropped the excess 20 pounds. Needless to say, we were both pretty impressed with the results.

Definition of Body Typing

The past several decades have seen encouraging glimmers of a North American shift from treating isolated symptoms (i.e. physical ailments, emotional issues, weight challenges) back to a more traditional model of looking at the whole person. Great strides have been made in understanding the ways a body can be strengthened in order to better allow correction of imbalances in areas such as weight management, energy and mood.

Unfortunately, however, while the same elements of achieving optimal health—proper dietary and water intake; correct amount and type of physical activity; sufficient sleep; and positive, stress-reducing, disciplined attitude—are needed for everyone, unless those elements are personalized to fit the unique characteristics of individuals, they simply will not work long term or for the majority. As Roger J. Williams, Ph.D., D.Sc, noted biochemical researcher from the University of Texas, stated:

> "If we continue to try to solve (nutritional) problems on the basis of the average man, we will be continuously in a muddle. Such a man does not exist."

A more recent and most welcome transition, therefore, has been the broader recognition of an individual's constitutional differences and unique dietary needs—a body typing concept that has been foundational to traditional Asian and Ayurvedic medicines for many generations.

There are many factors that determine body type, but it can be helpful to note the three primary body systems that shape an individual's unique biochemistry or body type:

**DIGGING DEEPER
Body Typing**

Interested in additional information on the long history of a body typing approach to good health? Check out: *Your Body Knows Best* by Ann Louise Gittleman; *The Metabolic Typing Diet* by William Wolcott and Trish Fahey; *The Nutrition Solution* by Harold Kristal, D.D.S. & James M. Haig, N.C.; and *The No-Grain Diet* by Dr. Joseph Mercola.

- ❏ The oxidative (metabolic) system—the rate and ease with which a body burns fuel.
- ❏ The autonomic nervous system—which of the brain components that control involuntary activities like digestion, heartbeat and immune system activity is more dominant, the Sympathetic/left brain or the Parasympathetic/right brain.
- ❏ The endocrine (glandular) system—influences exerted on metabolism by the body's secretion of different types of hormones.

The impact of these systems—particularly the oxidative system and the autonomic system—on the body is an integral part of the *KIB Body Type Survey* and, indeed, the *KIB* approach as a whole.

Because foods have particular influences on the body (i.e. stimulatory or inhibitory effects, acidic or alkalizing effects) it is helpful to choose foods that support the activity of your child's less dominant system (i.e. sympathetic or parasympathetic side of her autonomic system, or the fast or slow burning side of her oxidative system) in order to create a state that optimizes weight, energy and mental well-being. In simple terms, this means doing the *KIB Body Type Survey* (p. 179) with your child, and determining—of the three body types—which is that of your child. The next step is discovering and having her eat the optimal ratio or fuel mix of three key macronutrients—foods that are rich in protein (i.e. meats, nuts, seeds, legumes, dairy, seafood), foods that are rich in fat (i.e. butter, oils, nuts, nut butters, avocadoes) and foods that are rich in carbohydrates (i.e. grains, vegetables, fruits). In other words—personalizing an "Eating for Health" game plan.

Protein Body Types, those with a fast burning furnace or fuel burning system, do best when eating sufficient quantity of "logs"—foods that contain a high percentage of protein and healthy fats, and that take a relatively long time to be broken down and processed by the body. Intake of "kindling" or toothpick foods—carbohydrate foodstuffs that are broken down and processed by the body much more rapidly—should be carefully monitored and minimized. In order to reach optimum health, Protein Body Types require a food intake or fuel mix that has a higher percentage of protein-rich foods and fats as those food groups, among other benefits, do a better job in Protein Body Types of sustaining energy and balancing blood sugar levels.

Carbohydrate Body Types, on the other hand, do best when fuelling with a lower percentage of logs such as animal protein and fats, and a higher percentage of kindling foods such as vegetable proteins (i.e. legumes), vegetables, fruits and grains. Excess amounts of fat and protein, particularly heavier animal protein such as red meat, can leave Carbohydrate Body Types feeling physically sluggish and mentally lethargic.

Mixed Body Types will fall somewhere in the middle of the Protein and Carbohydrate Body Types and will reach optimal health on a fuel mix that includes relatively equal proportions of protein/fat and carbohydrate (i.e. grains, vegetables, fruit). With any body type, eating to keep balance in a body's strong points while strengthening weak systems is the ideal way to safely transition from obesity and ill health to a more balanced state of wellness.

What Are Key Body Type Differences?

As you will discover when your family members fill out the *KIB Body Type Survey*, body typing covers a wide range of physical and emotional characteristics. In brief, however, some of the main differences between body types are:

Food Favourites—While all body types have need for the full range of nutrients, different body types have varying needs with regard to type of macronutrients (i.e. protein from a meat or vegetarian source) and amount (i.e. a little healthy fat or more healthy fat). Some body types love meat and fattier foods; others prefer vegetables, fruits and grains.

Body Shape—Everyone has been created with a unique body shape. Even between several children that are carrying excess weight, some will have much thicker or denser bone or muscle, some will carry the extra weight around their abdominal area and some will have the extra weight distributed more evenly over their bodies.

Personality—Almost at birth, your child began to express her own personality and character. While each person will fall somewhere along the spectrum of personality traits, some body types tend to be more outgoing and seem almost to flourish on contact with others. Children of another body type prefer more time alone and have a quieter or shy personality.

Favourite Activities—Body types also differ in physical activity preference. Some body types really enjoy and thrive on regular physical activity while children of another body type may prefer more sedentary activity.

Organizational Style—Some body types have real skill in, and need for, organization. Children with another body type, however, may seem very disorganized or perhaps seem to have a very unique organizational style that other family members have not yet quite grasped!

Physical Energy—Some body types have low physical energy or energy peaks and dips, while others have high energy throughout the day.

Body Typing in Action

The first step to having your child eat according to her body type begins in **Find Your BALANCE** where you work with her to complete *KIB's Body Type Survey*, and determine whether your child is a Carbohydrate Body Type, a Protein Body Type or a Mixed Body Type. During **Find Your BALANCE**, all *KIB* kids follow a similar dietary plan, but once your child has moved into **Build Your BALANCE**, her intake of *KIB* food groups will be fine-tuned to be more in line with the ratio that is most appropriate for her body type—Protein, Carbohydrate or Mixed.

At its simplest, body typing is having your child's meals and snacks consist of the ratio of carbohydrate-rich foods (i.e. vegetables, whole grains, fruit), protein-rich foods (i.e. meat, poultry, seafood, dairy, nuts, legumes) and fat containing foods (i.e. avocadoes, butter, healthy oils) that leave her feeling satisfied and comfortably full; that sustain a healthy mood and energy level; and that allow her to more easily reach a healthy weight. Per recommendations found in *KIB's Fuel Mix Guidelines* (p. 187) and *Portion Size Guidelines* (p. 219) your child will learn to fill her plate in a manner that gives her the best possible sense of wellness.

And what exactly does that sense of wellness look like? Because food intake primarily affects us in three ways, how we feel 1-2 hours after eating should optimally produce positive responses in each of these three areas:

- ❑ Physically (i.e. energy, hunger, bloating).
- ❑ Emotionally (i.e. mood, patience, level of irritation).
- ❑ Mentally (i.e. mental clarity, sharpness, brain fog).

Evaluating body clues gives good indication whether or not the **quality** of your child's food—correct for her body type, whole food, free of added sugars and chemicals—and the **quantity** of her food—ratio of food groups, eating until comfortably full, not overeating—are the best fuel mix for her body. Until determining how she feels after a meal or snack becomes easy habit for your child, make use of *KIB's Food/Mood/Activity Log* (p. 211) and the *Fuel Mix Evaluation Chart* (p. 190). The *Food/ Mood/Activity Log* gives you room to record how your child feels after meals, snacks and exercise, and the *Fuel Mix Evaluation Chart* lists the way a body should feel after a correct intake of properly balanced food groups. It also lists the way a body feels after an incorrect intake of food groups or an intake of the wrong food groups for body type. This provides insight as to how your child should eat to correct any of her less than optimal responses.

Body Typing Tips for Parents and Kids

Because body typing is a somewhat unfamiliar concept for many people and is such a key concept of the *Kids in Balance* program, here are a few additional tips.

Things parents need to know about body typing:

Body Typing is Flexible—Rather than a rigid wellness formula, body typing is a way of listening to and responding to a body's unique characteristics and needs. The information given re: percentages of food group intake for each body type should be considered a guideline, not an exact blueprint.

Body Typing is Nothing New—Body typing has been practised in some form or other by a variety of cultures (i.e. Ayurvedic medicine, Traditional Chinese Medicine) for many centuries and is seeing recent North American interest and growing acceptance in complementary medicine, particularly in the past 50 years.

Body Typing Is Part of the Solution—Remember to set body typing on the foundation of other *KIB* nutritional principles. These principles will be discussed further under Food Intake Tools in chapter 11 but in brief, are:

- Utilize *KIB*'s **Food Pairing** principle. In order to satisfy the body's need for both volume and satisfaction in food intake, pair small amounts of denser foods such as protein-rich foods and fats that take longer to break down and provide the body with a sense of satisfaction, with larger amounts of foods that provide bulk and fibre such as raw and cooked vegetables. Depending upon body type and which of the three phases your child is in, you would also add in starchy vegetables, whole grains and small amounts of fruit.
- **Eat for Comfortable Fullness** but do not overeat. If your child is still hungry after her initial serving of body type appropriate protein-rich foods, vegetables, fats, whole grains and fruits, then serve a ¼ or ½ size second serving of the same body type appropriate foods.
- Start with **serving sizes based on the size of the hand**—your child's serving sizes based on her hand, your serving sizes based on your hand. Per *Portion Size Guidelines*, serve protein-rich foods sized to the palm of the hand and about ½-¾ inch [1-3 cm] thick; vegetables—raw and cooked—the size of two open hands; fat the size of the tip of your thumb to first knuckle; and starchy vegetables, whole grains and fruits the size of one clenched fist. Snacks would incorporate a protein-rich food and vegetables; a protein-rich food and fruit, or a protein-rich food, whole grain and vegetable, and would be ¼-½ the size of a meal serving.
- **Eat often**. All body types need to eat three meals per day. To keep from feeling excessive hunger, most children (and many adults) will also need to include several appropriate snacks throughout the day so they are not letting more than about 3-4 hours pass without eating.

Body Typing is Not a Make Work Project—Eating for body type does not involve making a separate meal for each family member. I have five children and have been eating this way for over 15 years. Much as my husband and I like to cook, we are not interested in making 63 meals a week (i.e. 3 meals a day, for seven days, for 3 different body types). Every body type needs a regular intake of vegetables and protein-rich foods, and once healthy weights are achieved, most family members will include at least one or two servings of starchy vegetables (i.e. sweet potatoes, yam, beets) or whole grains (i.e. quinoa, rice, sprouted bread) and probably at least one fruit each day.

For breakfast all body types can enjoy eggs and vegetables (see Tex-Mex Breakfast Eggs, p. 136) or smoothies (see Berry Coconut Milkshake, p. 177). Carbohydrate Body Types will also usually include a whole grain in the form of a toasted piece of sprouted grain bread or hot cereal. Protein Body Types may add turkey sausage to their eggs and need to determine at which meals they will have their starchy vegetable or whole grain choices.

If lunches are packed, it is easy to individualize for body type, or, if eaten at home, adjust per supper recommendations. Suppers can be based on foods that are common for all body types—protein-rich foods and vegetables—with Carbohydrate Body Types enjoying the white meat of a roast chicken and Protein Body Types going for the darker and more fatty thighs and drumsticks. Make meals such as taco salad and bean or beef burritos that can be individualized at the table. Adjusting recipes in the kitchen (i.e. dividing a stew in half and adding barley or potatoes to one half and leaving the other half a meat and vegetable combination) also keeps things simple.

Protein Body Types should include small amounts of some type of purine-rich foods on a daily basis. Purines are natural substances found in our cells and, to some degree, in most foods. Foods that contain concentrated amounts of purines, however, are particularly helpful for energy production in Protein Body Types. Purine-rich foods include: organ meats and certain types of seafood (i.e. liver, anchovies, sardines, caviar, shellfish, mackerel, herring, salmon, snapper, trout, tuna), red meats (i.e. beef, bison, lamb, pork, rabbit, venison), the darker meats of poultry (i.e. thighs, drumsticks) and certain vegetables and legumes (i.e. asparagus, green and yellow beans, cauliflower, celery, spinach, mushrooms, peas, kidney beans, lentils, lima beans, navy beans).

Things your child needs to know about body typing:

Every Body is Different—Your child has been designed with a one-of-a-kind personality, mind and body, and *KIB* encourages her to celebrate that wonderful uniqueness!

Every Body Has Strengths and Weaknesses—Body typing builds on your child's strengths and supports her areas of weakness. To help with your child's understanding of this concept, talk with her about the following question: "What do you already do well?" Is she great at remembering to drink water? Have her continue doing that. Does she already like a variety of vegetables? Keep her eating that variety and each week add a new type to try. Is kicking a soccer ball around at recess one of her favourite activities? Add that to her daily plan of activity. Does she have legs that are strong but move more slowly? Rather than attending the 100-yard dash try-outs, why not encourage your child to start power walking with mom or dad, or join her school's cross-country team? Does she have a positive attitude about life in general? Use that attitude to help her achieve the goals she has set in other important areas such as eating for health and getting to bed on time.

Every Body Has a Favourite Fuel Mix—Body typing helps you and your child learn how to fuel both for body type and for activity level. If your child is a Protein or Mixed Body Type she will soon understand that her snacks and meals will include more protein-rich foods and vegetables, and less whole grains and fruit. When she is in **Build Your BALANCE**, and has small amounts of starchy vegetables, whole grains and fruit back in her daily food intake, help your child recognize that one of the main roles of foods such as this is to provide energy for her body.

While a variety of factors influence the rate at which foods are digested (i.e. the body's supply of enzymes and hydrochloric acid, the ease with which a food's components are broken down, whether the food is eaten alone or in combination with other types of foods), in general, fruits and grains are digested more rapidly and are therefore available to provide energy for brain functioning and activity more quickly than proteins and fats. When your child eat grains and fruit, especially refined grains or sugars, and is then inactive for hours (i.e. does an evening couch potato routine), the extra blood sugar those grains and fruit give her is not used as fuel for exercise in the same way it would be if she had been more physically active. Instead the excess blood sugar supply is converted and stored as fat.

If your child is a Protein Body Type, have her enjoy appropriate amounts of starchy vegetables, grains and fruit, but be wise in when she eats them. The best option is to couple a small amount of protein-rich food with a serving of whole grains or fruit at times in the day when she will be engaging in movement, physical activity and exertion an hour or two following intake.

At this point, if you are reading the Body Type chapter for the first time, you can either continue with more in-depth Body Type information in *Fuel Mix Guidelines* (p. 187) or come back to those guidelines near the end of **Find Your BALANCE**. Regardless, realize by the time you have completed **Find Your BALANCE** and need to put additional body-typing information into practise, this component of the *KIB* approach will be clearer, and fall into place more easily.

KIB Stories for Life

I can't remember if I told you but her measurements were great!! She has certainly lost in every area!! She was very excited and it helps when family and friends are commenting on how "good" she is looking, not necessarily referring to her weight loss!

Belinda

B – Body Type 101

One Size Does not Fit All

Recognize that when it comes to dietary plans, one size does not fit all. What was good for Jack Sprat—no fat—did not sit at all well with his wife—who could eat no lean—and gives good indication that probably at least some of the Sprat children were Protein Body Types! We all have our own unique set of genes that translates into a unique rate of fuel burning and a need for a personalized ratio of essential nutrients.

KIB Body Type Survey

When you begin *KIB*'s personalized action plan, have your child complete *KIB*'s *Body Type Survey* and be prepared to follow *Fuel Mix Guidelines*. With scores in hand you will know which types and amounts of a wide range of healthy foods will provide your child with the best nutrients to sustain energy, enhance mental clarity and maintain healthy body weight.

Go Grocery Shopping

Regardless of your child's body type, you will need to lay in a supply of all the basics: meat, fish, dairy and eggs, legumes, nuts and seeds, lots of vegetables and at least a small selection of whole grains and fruit. As you fine-tune your child's dietary intake game plan you will discover which types of foods you need to buy more often and which you need in smaller amounts.

Partition Your Plate

Have your child divide her dinner plate (figuratively speaking) and then fill it with the right ratio of protein, fat and carbohydrate-rich foods for her body type. Getting the right volume and fuel-mix maximizes energy production and ensures that within 1-2 hours of eating, she will feel better than before she ate.

Monitor Your Responses

When food intake is matched to body type, three of the main ways your child's body has of communicating with her—appetite/cravings, energy levels and mental well-being—will all be sending resounding messages of "well done". If, however, your child experiences hunger or cravings, bloating, mental/physical lethargy, moodiness or diminished mental clarity she has probably eaten too much volume or the wrong ratio of foods. Adjust ratios or eliminate certain questionable foods for the next couple of meals and then re-evaluate.

Chapter 4

A - Attitude

Attitude is everything; choose a good one.

One of my favorite sayings
Seen in a newspaper advertisement almost 20 years ago

What *KIB* means by attitude is state of mind or, in a broader sense, the feelings, beliefs and values that determine actions. Both research and experience with *KIB* families show that how we look at a challenging issue such as excess weight has significant implications for what actions are taken and what results are realized. The feelings experienced about excess weight, the beliefs as to how that weight came to be, values about where the responsibility lies in tackling health challenges, and beliefs about our ability to deal with the weight all have an impact on the steps we take or do not take. In turn, those steps, or lack of steps, impact the outcome of our journey toward health.

Attitudes About What?

As you and your child journey through *KIB*'s 3-Phase Program, you will note at different points it is recommended that you take time to look at—and discuss in age-appropriate language—attitudes and beliefs about the following subjects:

Excess Weight—Some of the things to consider in a discussion about your child's extra weight are how it currently impacts his life and what differences your child thinks it will make when he is at a healthy weight. Always work to help your child understand that the extra weight is not the sum total of who he is and that you love him unconditionally, regardless of his physical condition. Be sure as well, to debunk a few prominent obesity myths (i.e. that your child cannot be physically fit if overweight, that being at a healthy weight means all your problems disappear).

Where the Extra Weight Came From—Often lack of knowledge can lead to a blaming mentality or a sense of impotence in being able to create change. As you and your child grow in understanding of the seven primary contributing factors to childhood obesity, you will find there is no need to blame people (i.e. family members who love to bake) or circumstances (i.e. genetics, finances) for the excess weight. You understand what has contributed to your child's excess weight and have a concrete game plan as to how you will tackle the challenge that extra weight presents.

Where the Responsibility Lies for Change—In the case of childhood obesity, there is much action that needs to take place. Schools, the medical profession, big business, grocery stores and government all have their roles in helping present accurate information, avoiding the undermining of good parental choices and supporting families who desire increased wellness. As you and your child accept the ultimate responsibility for your weight and health, however, along with that acceptance comes freedom from a victim mentality that could prevent you from feeling able to succeed. As you both recognize your part in where your child is today, you will both be on your way to owning the choices you can make for positive change.

Beliefs About Attempting the KIB Program—If you and your child believe you play no part in the excess weight he carries, and feel that change will be too hard, that there is nothing you can do to create health or that the process is not worth the effort, you will likely end up derailing your success before you even start the journey. Though the *KIB* program takes effort, it is simple, easy to follow and has a great track record. Other families—ones just like your family—have worked their way through the three *KIB* stages, enjoyed the food, cut their TV time, found new ways to exercise, learned fun family games, got to bed earlier, drank more water, and laughed and played their way to a healthier weight. There is virtually no reason why you and your child cannot do the same. It begins with how you think. Attitude is everything; you might as well choose a good one!

Whose Attitude?

So whose attitude am I talking about? When following the *KIB* program I suggest looking at the attitudes of three principle people/people groups:

- ❑ Your child's attitude. As a parent, you are best positioned to guide your child through lifestyle transition and therefore have an important role in modeling good attitude. Your child too, however, has to feel the need for change, grow in willingness to tackle new things and watch for negative self-talk or beliefs.
- ❑ Your family's attitude. Getting healthy is a family affair. The excess weight of a particular child may have been the impetus for your family's adoption of *KIB* principles but everyone will reap the rewards. Understanding the far-reaching benefits of a healthier lifestyle will positively affect each family member's results.
- ❑ The attitudes of those around you. Study after study[1,2] shows that the people we surround ourselves with have a great deal of impact on how we feel and the things we accomplish. Realize that many of the lifestyle changes you will be adopting are, to some degree, counter-culture. Be sure your circle of support includes positive people who believe in you and what you are doing. If appropriate, and your child is in agreement, talk with his teacher, coach or club leader. Let them know of the journey on which your child is embarking and give suggestions as to how they can help (i.e. offer non-sugared rewards for sports or academic achievement, be encouraging when they notice small steps of change).

Goals and Desires

Another crucial topic to cover before you and your child begin **Find Your BALANCE** is ensuring you both understand the differences between goals and desires. A key component of the *Kids in Balance* program is the discussion about and establishment of goals and motivators with your child. Understanding what motivates your child (i.e. one-on-one time with a parent, being able to purchase a better fitting or more flattering clothing item, having more energy for bike riding with friends) and setting reasonable, attainable goals (i.e. eating four servings of vegetables daily, walking around the block two times, trying one bite of a new supper side dish) make all the attitudinal difference between half-hearted effort and accountable, diligent perseverance. Those differences, in turn, set the stage for whether your efforts at the *Kids in Balance* program are yet another failed kick at the weight loss can or a very successful lifestyle change.

When parents and children begin the *KIB* program, they generally have a variety of longings. Some family members may hope for better concentration, most would like more energy and at least one—your child carrrying excess pounds—will want to reach a healthy balanced weight. Underlying the obvious longings there may also be subliminal wishes—that increased health and wellness will open the door to a sports or dance program for your child, create less tension around food choices or reduce schoolyard teasing and sense of frustration over excess weight's impact on wellness. Regardless of that inevitable swirl of conscious and subconscious thought, however, you can be sure that everything your family does, including starting the *Kids in Balance* program, represents an effort to reach a goal that somehow makes good sense to you and your child.

At times over the next few months you and your child may—OK, I will be frank, you **will**—feel discouragement and frustration and maybe even a little resentment and anger. Making concrete lifestyle change requires concrete action and sometimes that action, even if it is simple and easy, takes considerable dedication. As well, with change there are often emotional and psychological influences (i.e. cleanse symptoms) that heighten some of the normal physical reactions. Sometimes it may feel a little like a two-steps-forward-one-step-backwards expedition.

In an attempt to keep you and your child headed in the right direction I would like to pass on a foundational truth about goals that should make your path a little more straightforward. I first noted this truth in *The Marriage Builder,*[3] a book by psychologist Dr. Larry Crabb. Though, as the title indicates, the book is concerned with marriages, many of the points are relevant for other types of relationships and for life in general, including the information Crabb presents on the differences between goals and desires. The understanding of those differences can go a long way toward minimizing discouragement and maximizing attempts to achieve the goals you and your child will set over the next few months and beyond.

First, clearly recognize that when you and your child tackle **Find Your BALANCE** and are completing the *Setting Your Goals* worksheet (p. 214), I am talking about goals and not desires. Or in Crabb's words I am defining a **"goal as being an objective that is under your** [or your child's] **control and a desire as an objective that may legitimately and fervently be wanted** [by you or your child] **but that cannot be reached through your efforts alone."** When reaching an objective depends solely on your child's willingness to do certain things, it may properly be called a goal. A desire, on the other hand, requires the "uncertain co-operation of another" (Crabb) or even the uncertain cooperation of your child's body in the timing and rate at which it will shed excess weight. When determining your child's goals for pursuing increased health, think in terms of his own responses (i.e. walk for 15 minutes/3 times a week, follow the *KIB* **Find Your BALANCE** eating plan this week) rather than the responses of others or bodily responses that are somewhat outside his control (i.e. walk 3 times a week with a friend, shed 2 pounds this week).

What is the big difference you might say? Is it not just semantics? At first I wondered the same thing, but from personal and *KIB* family experience, I can say goals and desires are two decidedly different concepts, and knowing the difference goes a long way toward you and your child being able to achieve the things you want. Firstly, again with insight from Crabb, whether your child views an "objective as a goal or a desire makes a big difference in what [he] does with it." Your child's objective may be to lose five pounds in a week. If he sees his weight loss objective as a goal, he will try to find a way, perhaps even an unhealthy way, to make it happen. Because he does not, however, have the ability to completely determine whether or not his body will shed weight that week (i.e. increased activity levels could be increasing his lean tissue to fat tissue ratio and a higher amount of denser lean tissue could mean increased health and toning but little or no budging of the scale that week), there is a chance he could experience frustration, discouragement or anger.

Goals	Desires	What's the Difference?
I will walk for 30 minutes at least four times/week.	I want to drop two pant sizes in the next two months.	Your child has control over whether he takes the time to fit in a walk. He does not have control over how quickly his waist size will drop.
I will eat six servings of vegetables a day.	I hope to lose 35 pounds.	The rate at which your child loses weight requires the uncertain cooperation of his body. He can, however, control the amount of vegetables he eats.
I will be in bed by 10:00 PM each school night and 11:00 PM on weekends.	I want to feel less tired.	As your child chooses to get to bed on time, there is more likelihood of him gaining an increased level of energy. He controls the first, not the latter.

If you and your child have completed *KIB*'s *Goals and Motivators* worksheet accurately, any goals listed there will be able to be reached through your child's own efforts. And there, as Crabb reiterates, lies the difference: with proper goals your child is "responsible to act in ways that will realize [his] purpose." Some days he may not feel like taking the steps needed to achieve his goal (i.e. increase his water intake, eat a certain number of servings of vegetables, jump on the trampoline for 15 minutes), but he can do it if he chooses. By accomplishing his goals, there is a greater likelihood of your child reaching his desires (i.e. inch or fat loss), but even in a week when the desires do not happen, your child can be proud of his goal attainment and know that he has done the actions within his power to bring about the changes he would like to see happen.

Goals. Desires. Different words that require different actions. The proper way to handle a desire is with hope and faith. In Crabb's words, however, with a goal, "the proper response is a set of responsible actions." Work with your child to develop an attitude that has him set his heart on taking the small steps toward his goals and let the desires take care of themselves.

On the *Kids in Balance* journey it is important to know where you and your child are going. It is even more important the two of you know you are headed toward something you can actually accomplish. If your target is a desire, dream about, hope for or pray about it. If your target is a goal, then get to work and, with all the tools and support of the *KIB* program, reach that goal.

A - Attitude 101

Think You Can or Think You Can't?

Either way, you are probably right! While every component of *KIB*'s coaching program is important, in many ways attitude is key to them all. Changing the way you and your child think can be one of the most important factors in losing excess weight and gaining health. Attitude is everything; choose a good one.

Speak Truth in Where You Want to Be

Setting goals is an essential component of moving forward. Words we use, however, can either enhance or limit our ability to reach goals, so frame goals wisely and positively. Ensure goals your child sets are within reach and do not require the uncertain cooperation of another person or include factors he does not have complete control over (i.e. the rate at which his body will shed excess weight). Writing or speaking positively is also helpful: "We look forward to the increased energy a healthy lifestyle will provide." Or "We are having fun with the *Kids in Balance* program!"

Nix the All or Nothing Approach

Transitioning to better health takes time and involves process. In a challenging week where less than stellar lifestyle choices have been made remember the "yet" word: I did not eat 5 servings of vegetables a day, yet; our family bike ride did not happen, yet. Next week re-read your goals and go for them again.

Follow the Lead of the Experts

As to who to follow, look at people who are truly body, mind and spirit, full of health. Though a variety of elements contribute to wellness, there are a couple of consistent lifestyle factors in people that are free of disease, including the disease of obesity. The first is that most of them sleep well (see A Good Night's Sleep, p. 49). Secondly, people with good health generally have a good attitude. According to a wise but unknown author "Being in a good frame of mind helps keep one in the picture of health." Want good information? Pay attention to who is giving it and make sure the counsel you take comes from an encouraging, grateful and positive person.

Chapter 5

L – Laughter and Play

Smiling is my favorite exercise.

Author Unknown

As a concerned parent or caregiver reading this book, it is clear that you are taking childhood obesity seriously. You are doing your research and due diligence, and grabbing hold of the responsibility that goes along with the privilege of parenting. You are growing in your awareness of the many factors that impact a child's ability to reach and maintain a healthy weight. And finally, though I keep assuring you the *KIB* plan is simple and easy to follow, you grasp the concept that in order to best help your child achieve optimal wellness, you and she have some important work ahead of you.

Quite frankly, all that seriousness and responsibility might seem a little at odds with a childhood obesity solution entitled "Laughter and Play!" Not to worry. As previously mentioned, the *KIB* program is comprehensive, covering the seven primary contributing factors to childhood obesity. That means it tackles even less well-known factors, provided they have the research and results to back them up. Not sure if your humourous side is going to be able to rise to the occasion? Fortunately, and again as previously mentioned, the *Kids in Balance* program works best when tackled with teamwork. Optimum results happen when there is partnership between you as parent, the *KIB* material and your child. And luckily for parents, most children do quite well in the whole area of laughter and play.

More Laughter, Less Weight

A day without laughter can lead to a very dull weight loss plan. That is why the *KIB* approach takes into consideration research that has been done over the past couple of decades on laughter's ability to impact metabolism and calorie burning.

Several studies, including one by a team of researchers at Vanderbilt University in Nashville, Tennesee,[1] have looked at the energy expenditure of laughter. Results? Some likened the caloric burning capability of laughter to that of brisk walking,[2] and early laughter researcher, William Fry, an emeritus professor at Stanford University, has been credited with determining that 20 seconds of hard laughter gives the heart the same beneficial workout as three minutes of hard rowing.[3]

Lead researcher on the Vanderbilt University study, Maciej Buchowski, reported that participants burned up to 20% more calories when laughing than when not laughing. That means that a good solid 10-15 minutes of laughter per day could increase total daily energy expenditure by up to 50 calories. That might not seem like a lot, but over the course of a year that means a loss of about 4½ pounds. And 4½ pounds lost by a method that cost you virtually nothing, took very little time and was simple, easy and fun!

How All Work and No Play Make for Unhealthy Weight Levels

While laughter does indeed burn small amounts of calories, the main reason laughter plays a role in helping keep weight at a healthy level, however, is because laughter helps counteract the effects of stress in the body.[4] So what exactly does stress have to do with reaching and maintaining an appropriate weight? In a nutshell, stress increases levels of the hormone cortisol, a helpful hormone under certain circumstances and if kept in proper amounts. If cortisol levels become unnecessarily elevated or imbalanced, however, it is difficult to reach optimum weight and wellness.

To elaborate, cortisol—a fight or flight hormone produced by the adrenal glands—is a necessary hormone for particular types of situations. Its levels should be high in the morning to give your child a boost of energy to start her day. Or if your child was being chased by a tiger—an unlikely but highly stressful situation—she would appreciate the increased flow of glucose, protein and fat that cortisol would move out of her tissues for immediate use. As the day progresses, your child's cortisol level should take natural drops and then level slightly at different times until it reaches its lowest point at bedtime. Over the course of a proper, restful and deep sleep, her cortisol level increases to again reach a natural high at the beginning of the next day.

Because of today's heightened environmental and emotional stress levels, however, many people have elevated or imbalanced levels of cortisol and, therefore, are susceptible to conditions that high levels of the hormone are linked with:

- ❑ Food cravings.
- ❑ Storage of visceral fat (fat that surrounds abdominal organs).
- ❑ Diabetes.
- ❑ Insomnia.
- ❑ Heart disease.
- ❑ Lowered immune system functioning.
- ❑ Depression.

Because laughter has been shown to lower cortisol levels, as well as levels of several other stress hormones—epinephrine (increases your heart rate and energy levels, and elevates blood pressure) and dopamine (a component in the fight or flight response that also elevates blood pressure)[5]—it is clear that a couple of hearty belly chuckles or a joy-filled play session at the park can be very good tools in a weight loss plan.

Making Room for Play

So how exactly do you as a parent, manage to balance the very serious and responsible roles of financial provider, bill payer, household organizer, chauffer, teacher of values and guardian of the family faith, with the often down-played but equally serious and responsible role of family stress reliever? When job duties and home-front activities take up much of the day, is fitting in time for laughter and play even a possibility? Absolutely. It just takes a little shift in attitude.

First, follow the lead of your child. Statistics vary in their tallies as to how much kids and adults laugh, but without a doubt children laugh more each day than do grown-ups. Adults average 15-17 laughs a days and children more than 20 times that amount at 300-400 laughs per day. It makes sense then that your child helps set the tone for the degree of humor in the household. Ways you can follow along and increase your daily laughter quotient include:

Being Childlike—Playing board games, letting your child read you *Captain Underpants* books, and watching funny YouTube clips with your teen are all good ways to find the kid in a parent!

Being Spontaneous—Get out of a rut by trying a fun new recipe, taking advantage of freshly-fallen snow and a neighbourhood toboggan run, and letting your child wear her favourite outlandish outfit on your grocery shopping trip together.

Being Creative—To help spark creativity, give your child a silly but official-sounding kitchen job title and let your teen choose the music that accompanies her vegetable chopping task.

Being a Play Promoter—Recognize that though a primary parenting role is to help train up responsible adults, truly integrated and holistic adults value play and fun.

Secondly, let *KIB*'s *Day-at-at-Glance Guidelines* (p. 223) help put laughter and play in their rightful place in your household. Each day, under the Laughter and play section, there are recommendations for ensuring your household gets its daily quota of humor. And for that section, I encourage you to read ahead! Studies have shown that even the anticipation of laughter has the ability to increase levels of beta-endorphins—hormones that elevate mood—and human growth hormone—a hormone which plays many roles, including strengthening the immune system.[5,6] Just think, all that benefit merely from thinking about laughter and play. Does wellness get any simpler than that?

Relieving Stress Through Good Communication

Allowing for a little poetic license with an old saying, it seems clear that "The family that plays together stays together." As important a home harmonizer and stress-reliever as laughter and play, however, is a family system that allows for healthy communication patterns on every topic, not simply the funny ones. Next up, therefore, is looking at the ways your family communicates on topics such as discipline, beliefs and goals.

Healthy family communication is foundational to successful completion of the *KIB* program. Both your family's more formal communication **system**—whatever you call and how you lead your family meetings or "important talk" times—as well as your communication **style**—the ways in which your family discusses those far-reaching topics—are key factors in relieving stress, preventing misunderstanding and being able to handle challenging situations.

> **Re-Framing:**
>
> **Turning a comment away from the negative and into the positive.**

While healthy families greatly value the function that all members play in meetings, part of the important communication role that you as a parent play is to facilitate the tone, direction and manner in which family meetings occur. Of primary importance is that you are clear on the reasons for the meeting and have a method to help family members strategize ways to deal with any items or challenging issues that may be on the agenda. As a parent using the *KIB* approach, your role is to make your child's journey through this lifestyle transition as relatively smooth as possible. That entails working behind the scenes—and in front of them—to plan for and help your child navigate through a variety of challenges and triumphs while encouraging a healthy emotional balance—both yours and your child's!

Once you have a communication system in place (for additional tips see *Family Meeting Time—Communication Activity*, p. 207), you can begin to look at communication style. Here one of your primary strategies will be to use language that builds up rather than language that tears down. Helpful language that builds up is:

- ❑ Language that distinguishes self (or spirit or soul) from the body (physical).
- ❑ Language that is accepting of one's own unique characteristics.
- ❑ Language that chooses health and balance over appearance or measurement.
- ❑ Language that is free from negative comparisons that either elevate or diminish self.
- ❑ Language that shifts negative declarations into positive, realistic statements.

Language that Tears Down	Language that Builds Up	What's the Difference?
I want to be skinny.	I want to find my body's best state of balance.	Skinny is not most people's body type. Appropriate goal/desire language allows your child to set positive goals that are within her ability to reach and that are more in line with her own body's story.
I want to lose weight.	I want to lose unnecessary weight (i.e. excess fat).	You only want your child to take off the weight that puts her health at risk. If she moves into disordered eating and loses necessary weight (i.e. from muscles, organs), she increases other types of health risks.
I am on a diet.	I am changing to a healthier lifestyle.	This language will remind your child that this is not a "get-thin-quick" campaign. Rather than yo-yo dieting, your child is moving to the lifestyle best suited to her body.
It is not fair that other kids can eat sugary foods and stay skinny.	I will focus on my body's story and enjoy the success this focus will create in my life.	By encouraging your child to focus on her unique body story, focus will move from being a victim to having control.

When you open discussion about various aspects of the *KIB* program, encourage your child to speak honestly about her thoughts and feelings. An open talk about the challenges of dealing with obesity and the positive solutions before you has the potential to set you both free from the feelings of shame and avoidance that often accompany an overweight condition. While there may be tears and a range of emotions expressed, discussion of this type is an ideal time for you to show your child how to re-frame negative thoughts. Re-framing means allowing your child to express how she feels but to then help her see beyond how she feels. While negative thoughts are not dismissed or stuffed, they can usually be viewed in another, more positive light (i.e. seeing a glass half full as opposed to half empty). Even very discouraging situations can be re-framed with an evaluation of what contributed to the situation and the encouraging possibility of making different choices in the future.

Making positive language choices protects your child's sense of self-esteem by providing healthy guidelines for her thoughts. For instance, steering your child away from thinking there is only one ideal body weight or body type; protecting her from embracing fad or disordered eating; and pointing her toward acceptance of her unique story, are all helpful language choices which will support a healthy lifestyle. With *Kids in Balance*, your child will learn what she can do to get and keep her body in its healthiest state, while you help ensure that practical information is presented and interpreted by your child in a sound manner.

As you begin **Find Your BALANCE**, the *KIB Day-at-a-Glance Guidelines* will help move you and your child toward an increased amount of laughter and play in your household, and to ensuring there is health, positiveness and lightness in the way you and your child communicate about even very challenging issues. Each of those small steps can go a long way to providing the calm, joyous and relatively stress-free environment that promotes optimum wellness for you and your child.

Planning
As with sports, so often goes life:

"Players who have spent time thinking about and developing a game plan to use for the key points in a match are much more likely to find success when they are faced with a pressure situation. Having a pressure point game plan is often the key to winning the big points and pulling out the close matches."

Mike Uretsky
Tennis player/coach

KIB Stories for Life

We also tried the vegetable "Jicama" for the first time yesterday. Meaghan and I both LOVED it!! Meaghan says it tastes like an apple. This is great for us, as you know I'm a hard one to please in the veggie category! Talk to you again. Must get on that treadmill!

Naomi

L – Laughter and Play 101

Control Cortisol Production

It would be naive to think that simply laughing more each day is enough to bring cortisol production into its proper place. Regular daily routines of sleep/wake patterns, meal times, physical activity and quiet times are essential, as is appropriate nutritional intake—particularly of protein, B vitamins, essential fatty acids (EFAs), calcium and magnesium. Most children benefit from taking a high quality daily multivitamin and EFA supplement (see *KIB-Friendly Supplements* p. 196) to ensure all their nutritional needs are being met but laughter and play, however, perform an important role and should be a regular part of daily stress-busting routines as well.

Have You Heard the One About . . .

Researchers tell us that 10-15 minutes of laughter burns about 50 calories. Let's see, increased metabolism and calorie burning just for watching reruns of The Simpsons or reading an Archie comic? Maybe listening to your child's favorite Knock Knock joke one more time makes sense!

Real vs. Canned

Laughter does not mean denial. I firmly believe in recognizing the problem of childhood obesity and engaging in purposeful activity to tackle that problem. The serious effort lifestyle and attitude change requires cannot be minimized. It is both reasonable and helpful, however, amidst concerted effort in tackling a difficult situation, to have bouts of joy and levity. They give a needed break, enhance and encourage the spirit and remind the whole family that there is life after broccoli! And while spontaneous laughter is likely the most fun, even working at making yourself laugh can be effective. Researchers found that forced laughter too was able to produce some of the positive effects of a genuine response[7] to things like a brilliant pun, excellent joke of the day or top-notch slapstick.

And If That Wasn't Enough

Laughter has been found to produce far-reaching effects beyond impact on cortisol levels and energy expenditure. Laughter has also been shown to lower blood pressure, increase muscle flexion and trigger release of endorphins, our body's natural painkillers and enhancers of our sense of well being. By increasing antibodies and natural killer cells, laughter also boosts functioning of the immune system.

Chapter 6

A - Activity

A bear, however hard he tries, grows tubby without exercise.

Pooh's Little Instruction Book
Inspired by A. A. Milne

While there are varying opinions on the degree and types of activity required for healthy weight loss and maintenance, there is almost universal acceptance of the fact that exercise in some form is needed to reach optimal health and wellness. Before encouraging your child to lace up his runners, however, it is important to understand the different types of activity and the role that each plays in helping your child reach a healthy weigh.

Three Essential Types of Exercise

In the *KIB* program, I advocate increasing activity slowly and building on your child's fitness strengths. Eventually, however, you will want your child's physical activity to incorporate three primary types of exercise:

Functional Fitness—This term describes exercise that occurs as part of a normal day's activities. More formally known as NEAT—non-exercise activity thermogenesis—functional fitness describes the energy expended for everything we do that is not sleeping, eating or sports-like/planned exercise[1]. Functional fitness is one of the simplest places for families to increase daily activity levels: it builds on already occurring actions, costs little in terms of time and money, requires no special equipment and means your child can use already acquired abilities. What does that look like on a day-to-day basis? Park farther from the mall entrance when you and your child go on a shopping trip; take the stairs instead of the elevator; have your child take a short stretch break or a walk around the yard between tackling sections of homework; re-arrange the chore list to give your child more physically active responsibilities such as cleaning the garage; and, if safe, instead of giving him a ride, have your child walk to school or friends' houses. For best health results, your child should work toward making functional fitness a regular and increasing part of his life.

Longer Duration/Moderate Intensity Exercise—Whenever your child joins you on the tennis court, briskly walks the dog, takes swimming lessons, bike rides with a friend or plays community soccer, he participates in a second important type of exercise, that which is of a moderate intensity but which can be sustained for a longer period of time. This type of aerobic activity burns calories at a lower rate than higher intensity activity, but because your child can sustain it for greater duration, the potential is there to expend more energy. While functional fitness too brings with it some degree of increased calorie burning, the additional benefits of aerobic activity include an increased supply of oxygen to the blood, and increased endorphins—your body's natural painkillers. As well, aerobic activity enhances immune system function. Work with your child to incorporate longer duration/moderate intensity exercise 2-3 times/week.

Shorter Duration/Higher Intensity Exercise—Exercise of this type is done for 15-20 minutes, 2-3 times/week, and alternates a short work cycle (i.e. intense activity) with a rest cycle (i.e. a time to recover). Interval intensity exercise causes the body to burn fat at a higher rate for several hours after the workout; increases lung volume; strengthens the cardiovascular system; preserves lean tissue; stabilizes blood sugar levels; improves muscle tone; firms skin—a real benefit when a child experiences significant weight loss; and increases production of Human Growth Hormone (which in turn produces a variety of positive benefits including better sleep, stronger bones and muscles, enhanced disease resistance and more positive moods). Other benefits of interval exercise are that it can easily be adapted to many types of kid-friendly activity, is relatively easy to fit into a busy family schedule, and children and teens generally love the aspect of moving from resting to working pace throughout the activity. Head off on an interval intensity power walk with your child or simply have him do a 15-minute swim where he alternates a very fast lap with a very slow lap. Whichever interval exercise activity you and your child decide upon, you will get a lot of benefit for a relatively small amount of time and effort.

On Your Mark, Get Set, Go!

While understanding the value of different types of exercise is important, when childhood obesity is the challenge, the first question with regard to physical activity is often, "Where do we begin?" If your child does virtually no exercise, then the place to start is with increased functional fitness. Overweight children often feel physically or emotionally uncomfortable engaging in strenuous activity. Begin, therefore, by incorporating simple, daily activities such as walking to school or the library, more rigorous household chores, using a bike for shorter errands, mowing the lawn or playing a game of croquet with mom or dad. As body and mind comfort levels improve, step up physical exercise. Watch for the signs—small weight loss, interest in a new activity, improved energy—that say your child is ready to move to an increased level of activity. Set clear expectations on the value of physical exercise and the need for a sufficient amount of activity to become a regular part of life, but allow flexibility in how that value is expressed.

Once your child has increased his levels of functional fitness or if he is already a naturally active child, next look at increasing longer duration/moderate intensity exercise and shorter duration/higher intensity exercise. If your child wants to sign up for a community sports team, join a dance troupe or take a martial arts class, then by all means follow his lead and start with the longer duration/moderate intensity exercise. If, however, he has no preference, because shorter duration/higher intensity exercise takes less time and produces fairly quick physical responses, I would suggest starting there.

While there are several different programs patterned on the shorter duration/higher intensity type of exercise, I particularly like the PACE plan[2] developed by anti-aging physician, nutritionist and researcher Dr. Al Sears. I find his approach resonates well with children and teens, is simple to understand and can be easily incorporated in a variety of fun ways. In real life, that means having your child pick one of his favorite aerobic activities (i.e. biking, walking, jumping on the trampoline) and commit to incorporating shorter more intense periods of that activity into his schedule every couple of days. Have your child start with several minutes of slower warm-up activity and then alternate 6-8 cycles of work (i.e. 30-60 seconds of very speedy walking) with 6-8 cycles of rest (i.e. 60-90 seconds of very slow walking). After the last work cycle, have your child end with a couple minutes of cool down activity (i.e. slower walking and stretching). Alternating 1-minute work/1-minute rest periods is a simple place to start.

Once your child has the alternating work and rest cycles down pat, he can move toward the progressive part of the PACE program by, over the course of a PACE workout, gradually shortening the length and increasing the intensity of his work cycles. For example, if he is "PACEing" a 20 minute bike ride, he would keep his rest periods consistent—say 2 minutes—but progressively move toward shorter work periods—from 2 or 3 minutes at the start of the activity to a 30 second final work period. As your child shortens the length of his work periods, he would simultaneously increase each work period's intensity. That means that while his first work period may be only slightly faster than his rest periods, by the time he gets to his final 30-second work period, he will be peddling pretty darn fast!

In addition to the exercise basics, here are several more important exercise tips:

❑ While functional fitness, longer duration/moderate intensity exercise and shorter duration/higher intensity exercise should be incorporated early in a child's life and stay with him as a lifelong pattern, as your child passes through puberty and reaches his later teen/young adult years, there are a couple of other important types of exercise to incorporate as lifestyle. The first is some program of muscle toning/flexibility exercise such as Callanetics (my favourite!), Pilates or the more familiar sit-ups, crunches and squats. Secondly, he will likely want to add in some form of strength-building exercise such as a mild weight-training program. Among other benefits, the toning/flexibility exercise keeps muscles firm and lengthened, and the strength-building exercise builds strong bones. While there are differences of opinion as to what age is best to begin a strength-training program, research seems to indicate that strength training can begin when puberty has started. The key is to learn from someone certified in this form of exercise, to start with light loads and to use proper technique.

❑ Recognize that different body types often view exercise differently. Whereas Carbohydrate Body Types and most Mixed Body Types often enjoy or feel a strong need to exercise, some Protein Body Types may consider exercise nothing more than work, and unpleasant work at that. For Protein Body Types whose exercise attitude could use a shift, be sure to encourage high levels of functional fitness and to incorporate other types of exercise in a form that draws on what is more often a primary interest of this body type—social or group interaction. Children with a Protein Body Type may prefer to get their exercise playing street hockey with neighbourhood kids or on a sports team of some type. Teenaged Protein Body Types may be open to taking a jazz or hip-hop class or getting a couple of friends to join them in a local water aerobics program. That way, the exercise comes as a natural side-benefit of a primary characteristic Protein Body Types often have—the enjoyment of engaging in an easy-going manner with a wide range of friends.

❑ Regardless of the type of exercise, always increase activity levels gradually. Allow for exercise days and rest days. As well, keep your child well hydrated and be sure your child's doctor has approved an active exercise program.

Inactivity

And finally, a chapter on the role of **activity** in health and wellness would not be complete without a note on the role of **inactivity** in health and wellness. Over the last 30-40 years, there has been a marked decrease in functional fitness or NEAT, the calories burned due to all activity beyond sleeping, eating and formalized exercise. Changes such as our type of daily chore activity; degree of sedentariness in jobs; use of vehicles for even trips of short duration; reduction or elimination of physical education courses and playground time in schools; and the increased level of TV viewing, have produced small shifts in our energy expenditure each day that have led to huge shifts in our level of excess body weight. Having your child add planned exercise and activity to his life is important, but I cannot emphasize enough the role of functional fitness—converting more of your child's inactive moments each day to moments of even slightly increased activity— in reaching and maintaining a healthy weight.

<table>
<tr><td>

DIGGING DEEPER
Inactivity

For an informative and creative look at the effects of the past couple of decades worth of small, more sedentary, lifestyle shifts download the Center for Consumer Freedom's report, *"Small Choices, Big Bodies"* (www.obesitymyths.com /downloads/SCBB.pdf). While I do not agree with all of the views of the Centre for Consumer Freedom, they have done an excellent job of compiling information as to the significant role that increased inactivity has played in today's obesity epidemic; their report is well worth a read.

</td><td>

One of the primary places you can have effect with your child in the area of decreasing inactivity is in reducing the amount of his screen time. According to Nielsen Media Research, in 2006 Americans reached the fairly amazing statistics of having more television sets than people in the average American home and increased viewing time to almost two months of every year. Unfortunately, we did not stop there. In the first quarter of 2010, statistics showed Americans averaged the following time weekly: 35 hours, 34 minutes watching television; approximately 2 hours timeshifting (making use of the option to watch a TV show in an alternate timeslot); 3 hours, 52 minutes using the Internet; 20 minutes watching online video; and 4 minutes watching mobile video.[2] That is a heck of a lot of screen time!

And unfortunately, it seems the effects of TV watching are not as simple as a lack of calorie burning during your child's period of inactivity (and I do mean inactivity; TV watching burns just slightly more calories than sleeping). Evidence indicates that watching television also impacts metabolic rate in general, not simply during the time spent viewing a show. In other words, if your child accumulates a lot of screen time compared to a child who makes only occasional use of screen time, your child will burn fewer calories than the child with less screen time, even if they have the same degree of physical activity.

As most families are unlikely to totally rid their home of all TVs and computers—and cell phones have become the norm for most teens—the key is wise monitoring to keep the screen monster at bay. To follow are a few suggestions:

</td></tr>
</table>

- Keep the TV off before school and during meal times.
- Have a "no screens on in the house" hour each day (i.e. no TV, no computers or video games) and use the time for reading, a family game or listening to music—and remember, toe tapping is a great form of functional fitness!
- Pre-plan TV viewing rather than randomly channel surfing (i.e. allot a certain amount of daily screen time for your child and together determine when that time will be used).
- Increase the activity level of your screen time (i.e. make Wii-Fit your video game of choice, jump on a rebounder while watching your favourite show, do jumping jacks during commercials).
- In good weather, cut screen time further to allow for more outdoor play.
- Have your child balance activity with inactivity (i.e. accumulate 30 active play minutes to trade in for 15 minutes of screen time).

Television, computers and cell phones are likely here to stay. Use them in moderation, however, and rather than a health impediment, they can keep their role as helpful tools.

KIB Stories for Life

We're back on track for the New Year and despite it all managed to keep some control over Christmas or better than I feared. Meaghan gained back 1 pound and I gained back 4 pounds, but I expected that. Meaghan has grown yet again, so that would explain some of it and we did deviate off healthy eating for a few weeks.

I know for sure that Meaghan has gained confidence in herself since she has slimmed down. People who haven't seen her in a while are overwhelmed at how wonderful she looks and this is positive feedback that has enabled her to be more confident in how she acts and talks. She tells me about the choices she makes and is very aware of them. Your program couldn't have come at a better time for her in her development stage. I now see so many kids of her former size and wish they could go on your program and learn what we have.

Best wishes for a successful New Year . . . you offer a wonderful program to families!

Take care,
Naomi

A – Activity 101

Talk to Your Health Care Professionals

Before beginning a new exercise program, have your child seen by relevant health care practitioners (i.e. doctor, chiropractor).

Slow But Steady Wins the Race

While physical activity is an essential component of weight loss, pushing your child too quickly into more intense exercise or into activities that he really does not enjoy can lead to physical injury or emotional angst. In a family meeting, discuss the fact that fitness has become a family priority and then lead by example and encouragement.

Do More of What you Already Do

Does your child already enjoy swim class or jumping on the trampoline? Add a session of diving to his swim program and join him for extra time on the trampoline each day. If family bike rides are the norm, find a steeper route to increase intensity or pack additional water and lengthen the distance a bit.

Mix Things Up

Though there are different opinions on how to best increase lung capacity, strengthen the heart and burn fat, as mentioned, I especially like the PACE method developed by Dr. Al Sears (www.alsearsmd.com/category/fitness). Start a simplified version of PACE by doing 20 minutes of an activity (i.e. biking, trampoline, walking) 2-3 times/week. Include a couple of minutes of warm up and a couple of minutes of cool down. Between warm up and cool down, do short bursts of intense activity (i.e. a work phase of 2 minutes initially that gradually decreases to 30 seconds while you up the intensity). Intersperse the work phases with a couple minutes of rest—recovery time. Hmmm, lots of different activities, varying paces and intensities, a short work out; sounds like Kick the Can, Frozen Tag, a fun hilly bike ride or playing "Jaws" at the local pool—activities a kid and parents could really enjoy!

Get an Early Start

Exercise is so important that fitting it in wherever it works is a priority but consider slotting it in first thing in the morning. There are metabolic reasons—less glucose in the bloodstream to interfere with fat burning for one—but perhaps equally important is the sense of accomplishment and satisfaction at having already engaged in physical activity for the day.

Chapter 7

N – A Good Night's Sleep

For participants who sleep less than eight hours a night—74 percent of the group—
BMI was inversely proportional to sleep duration. That is, the less sleep
a subject got, the greater the person's BMI and thus the more overweight.

Tufts University Health & Nutrition Letter, 2005[1]

Over the last number of decades, the amount of sleep experienced each night, by both adults and children, has been in decline. Blame it on the fact many of us take on too many daily tasks to allow for a reasonable amount of shuteye each night and the availability of late-night or even all-night activities such as shopping, movie and television viewing, drive-through restaurants and Internet access. Regardless of cause, however, the fact remains that we are going to bed later and garnering fewer hours of deep, restful sleep.

Why Sleep is Important

Research has shown that accumulated sleep deprivation contributes to a variety of physical and mental problems, including:

- ❑ Increased rate of accidents (i.e. on the job, vehicle).
- ❑ Impaired immune system functioning.
- ❑ Disrupted hormone release.
- ❑ Reduced ability to deal with stress.
- ❑ Diminished mental clarity.
- ❑ Impaired memory.
- ❑ Higher rates of depression.

More closely related to the reason you are reading this book, however, quality sleep also appears to be an important factor in reaching and maintaining a healthy weight. Studies in both animals and humans show consistent correlation between ongoing insufficient amounts of sleep and excess body fat.[2]

How Less Sleep Leads to More Weight

So how exactly does a smaller amount of sleep lead to one carrying larger amounts of excess weight? While it does not happen overnight—most studies indicate the sleep deprivation needs to be longer term—there seem to be several factors at play in the link. One of the primary reasons for the excess weight was seen in a study showing participants that experienced sleep curtailment had increased levels of hunger.[3] Increased appetite can definitely contribute to obesity, especially if, as occurred with the study participants, the hunger cravings were not for healthy protein-rich foods, fresh vegetables or even fruit but rather sweets, starchy foods and salty snacks.

DIGGING DEEPER
Sleep—Getting Enough

For more information on returning to the sleep patterns that produced health and wellness generations ago, check out *Lights Out* by T.S. Wiley and Bent Formby, Ph.D. It contains great suggestions on how to gain health by sleeping in sync with nature.

Another reason for insufficient sleep leading to excess weight is the reality that an inadequate supply of deep rest can lead to more stress. As noted in the **Attitude** chapter, increased stress means increased cortisol production by the adrenal glands. That, in turn, can lead to increased accumulation of fat, in particular, abdominal fat.

Additionally, shortened sleep duration impacts circadian rhythms—the ranges of physiological and behavioural characteristics that are predominately controlled by an individual's biological time clock. Circadian rhythms are also, however, highly influenced by the light/dark cycles that naturally occur in each 24-hour period. Because those rhythms have a role in hormonal balance, both hormone production and regulation are affected by sleep.

Leptin, a hormone that works to decrease appetite, and ghrelin, a hormone that increases feelings of hunger, are both impacted by insufficient sleep.[4] As leptin secretion largely occurs during sleep, its levels are reduced with inadequate amounts of sleep. Ghrelin production, on the other hand, increases with insufficient amounts of sleep. What that means for your child is that if she consistently gets insufficient amounts of sleep, she is likely to experience an increased sense of hunger that can lead to overeating.

Sleep loss has also been shown to impact the body with regard to glucose tolerance,[5] the ease with which the body is able to regulate blood sugar levels by secreting proper amounts of insulin. Because lack of sleep can lead to decreased glucose tolerance, and that condition is a risk factor for obesity, insufficient sleep can take another direct hit—once again, metabolically—on your child's ability to reach and maintain a healthy weight.

Where Did Your Child's Sleep Time Go?

While it is likely that your child is involved to a greater degree in structured activities than you were as a child, with today's labour-saving devices and vehicle usage, she is also probably spending less time on chores such as washing dishes, mowing the lawn or walking to the corner store for eggs or bread. What then is cutting into her sleep time? If you want to look seriously at the correlation between obesity and sleep, it is well worth spending time examining the link between sleep and screen time—the amount of time spent texting, and viewing televisions, computers and video games. As these devices have become many children and teens' favourite electrical appliances, evaluating their healthfulness on a number of levels, including obesity, makes common sense.

We have already taken a look at the first likely link between screen time and obesity with the activity vs. inactivity factor examined in the **Activity** chapter. To reiterate, if your child is watching TV, surfing the net or texting her friend, she is not riding a bike, playing soccer, doing a paper route, climbing a tree, joining in a board game or walking on the dock at the beach. Bottom line, every minute spent watching a screen means one less minute of being in motion.

If your child is watching more TV, however, it is most likely coming not only at the expense of activity but also of sleep. An article[6] on the Avon Longitudinal Study of Parents and Children (ALSPAC)—a study that included more than 14,000 participants—lists eight primary factors the research found to influence childhood obesity, sleep duration being one of those factors. Among the circumstances found to be most significant in determining the amount of sleep a 7-year old child got each night was the amount of time a child spent watching television.

TV time is impacting older children and teens as well. For a number of years, it seemed time spent TV viewing was diminishing in adolescents, likely due to an increased usage of computers, video games and digital music players. In 2005, however, according to Nielsen Media Research, that usage took an upturn again but this time as a result of later night and early morning TV viewing. Unfortunately if your teen is watching TV at that time of the day or night it means duration of sleep is almost certainly being eroded.

Suggestions for a Good Night's Sleep

If your child is already getting adequate sleep each night (i.e. while children vary in their sleep needs, usual recommendations are 10 hours for children, 9 hours for teens), congratulations! You are well on your way to having this facet of *KIB*'s healthy weight management approach under control. If, however, your child could use a little help in the sleep department, please make getting her to bed on time a priority. It is very difficult to shed excess weight while being in a constant sleep deficit.

Over the years, I have come across, used, and recommended a variety of suggestions for a better night's sleep. And for most people, the standard list is often helpful:

- ❑ Go to bed and get up at the same time each day.
- ❑ Avoid heavy meals before you go to bed.
- ❑ Keep intense exercise a couple of hours away from bedtime.
- ❑ Make use of "white noise" (i.e. turn on a small fan as gentle, consistent background noise).
- ❑ Avoid caffeine (i.e. found in chocolate, caffeinated soft drinks, coffee and many teas).
- ❑ Take a hot bath before bed.
- ❑ Ensure bedroom is dark (i.e. optimizes melatonin production, a sleep-enhancing hormone).
- ❑ Write a "to do" list to keep yourself from needlessly reviewing those items.

While **quantity** of sleep is important, more recently, however, with the advent of wide spread use of television, computers, cell phones and other electronic equipment, there are a few additional factors to consider with regard to **quality** of sleep.

EMFs and Sleep

Electro-magnetic frequencies (EMFs) are invisible electrical energy waves surrounding any electrical device. They are created whenever electricity is generated or used. All the helpful tools that we have so come to love—coffee pots, power saws, copy machines, blow dryers, dishwashers, cordless phones—to say nothing of the power lines, transformers and electrical wirings that provide the "juice" for our favourites to function, are now emitting EMFs which are estimated to be 100 million times greater than that of a hundred years ago. The ever-growing field of wireless technology has also contributed to a significant proliferation of EMFs. Enough so that many researchers are wondering if the convenience of a cell phone, PDA, Bluetooth or laptop Internet connection on every street corner could be coming at a steep health and wellness price.

Not every scientist and health professional believes EMFs pose a health risk, however, and if you do much research at all you will see that many experts feel that limited, non-chronic exposure to EMFs is not dangerous. So if even a variety of authorities in this field do not seem to care about EMFs, why should you be concerned about any potential connection between EMFs and obesity?

Firstly, because even if limited non-chronic exposure to EMFs proves to be safe, with the widespread use of cell phones and degree of businesses and schools going wireless, very few of us currently experience EMF exposure to that minor degree. Rather, most of us receive fairly intense and/or fairly repetitive exposure. The complex rhythms with which our cells and atoms transfer energy and information, and our biofield—a term coined by the US National Institute of Health (NIH) that refers to the outward extension of that energy and information—can be disturbed and disrupted by EMFs. The resultant responses in our body (i.e. hardening of cell membranes, cellular fatigue, reduced ability for cells to take in nutrients and rid themselves of toxins) can contribute to a wide range of health challenges such as headaches, fatigue, disturbed moods and nervous system functioning, and immune system compromise. More specifically related to sleep and obesity, EMFs can also contribute to hormonal disruption and insomnia.

And secondly, attention to EMFs may be warranted because not all health practitioners are unconcerned with EMFs. Leading health expert and author, Dr. Andrew Weil, believes that "electromagnetic pollution (EMF) may be the most significant form of pollution man has produced in this century, all the more dangerous because it is invisible and insensible." Even the generally conservative World Health Organization's recent statement introducing its EMF Report[7] shows caution: "The World Health Organization (WHO) takes seriously the concerns raised by reports about possible health effects from exposure to electromagnetic fields (EMF). . . .**EMF has become one of the most pervasive environmental influences and exposure levels at many frequencies are increasing significantly** as the technological revolution continues unabated and new applications using different parts of the spectrum are found shows the need for further exploration of this topic."

Therefore, in addition to the previously listed good night sleep tips, here are a couple of EMF suggestions to help ensure a higher quality of sleep:

- ❑ Increase your child's distance from EMF sources. Since magnetic fields often significantly drop off within 3 feet of the source, remove computers, digital clocks and cell phone chargers from your child's bedroom.
- ❑ Encourage texting over cell phone calling. While the cell phone will still be close to your child's body, it will be farther removed from her brain.
- ❑ Remove cell phones from your child's room at night. EMFs aside, keeping cell phones out of your child's room is a good idea simply to avoid the sleep disruption that can occur because of incoming text messages. Having had five teenagers, I can also speak to the fact that having your child's cell phone stored overnight in a location other than her bedroom

means her desire to immediately connect with her closest friends ensures she gets up in a timely fashion!

- ❑ Avoid screen time just before bed. Whether it is due to the brain stimulation, increased stress levels because of the type of television show being watched or some component of the impact of EMFs on the body, television before bed has been shown to negatively impact sleep patterns. Instead implement bedtime routines that include reading, listening to quiet music, goodnight prayers or a pleasant family chat.

And lastly, keep the television out of your child's bedroom. Period. There are likely a variety of reasons contributing to the fact that studies[8,9] show children with TVs in their rooms have up to 30% more chance of being obese than their peers. Regardless of the underlying cause, however, that is too high a statistic to ignore.

KIB Stories for Life

Hannah is continuing to have success with the lifestyle change. Her friend's mom commented on how she makes smart choices when over for dinner, and has turned down many bad choices on her own.

Jeannie

N – A Good Night's Sleep 101

Set and Keep an Appropriate Bedtime

The refreshment and restoration that comes to a body during a good night's sleep is essential to wellness. Most older children and teens need 9-10 hours sleep per night, and changing sleep/wake-up times can disrupt body rhythms. Therefore set a reasonable and regular bedtime and waking time for your child and ensure they are kept.

Establish a Bedtime Routine

Preparing mind, body and soul for bedtime is key to ensuring a restful sleep. The age and personality of your child will determine routines but suggestions include a warm bath, story time/personal reading, a quiet family game, fresh air, a chat with mom and/or dad and a snack (a small amount of protein and fruit can help with melatonin and serotonin production). As well, to add to sleep time peace, rather than carrying problems over to the next day, make it a habit to find resolution to conflict before bedtime.

Lights Out

In days gone by, sunset and the resulting growing darkness signaled the body to produce adequate amounts of melatonin, a hormone that helps with many functions including sleep. Today's growing levels of light pollution mean most of us sleep in rooms backlit by street lamps, digital alarm clock glow or nightlights. In order to have melatonin production at optimum levels, ensure your child's room is as dark as possible at night. Place room-darkening shades on windows, swap the digital clock for a battery one where the numbers are not lit up, and move the nightlight to the hallway where it can provide washroom direction without creating light in your child's room.

Minimize EMFs

Because of their smaller, less dense bones and growing bodies, children and teens can, (even more than adults) be negatively impacted by the electrical pollution produced by electrical appliances and electronic wireless devices. Clear your child's bedroom of computers, cell phones and cordless landlines; avoid electric blankets and water beds; and revert to a battery operated alarm clock. EMFs negatively impact melatonin production that, in turn, can lead to myriads of health challenges—sleep disturbance is one of them.

Chapter 8

C – Clean Water

Water is the most neglected nutrient in your diet but one of the most vital.

Kelly Barton

If a child carrying excess weight did nothing but increase his water intake and eliminate every additional type of beverage (i.e. pop, diet pop, juice, juice beverages, coffee, regular tea) other than perhaps an optional glass of milk per day, he would almost certainly lose weight and gain health. Having water be your child's beverage of choice goes a long way to cleansing and balancing body systems. Then the body can start processing foods more efficiently and effectively, and begin the process of releasing stored fat.

What Exactly is Clean Water?

Your mom was right—drinking 8-12 glasses of water a day is a great idea. What she might not have told you, however, is that while the amount of water intake is important, the quality of the water also plays a factor in the health you and your child will experience.

Even in your grandparents' day, drinking water was never pure. The lake or river our ancestors used as their water source inevitably contained leaves, animal waste and other natural material. Today, however, a glass of water containing only decaying vegetation looks pretty good. How's that? Mainly because a glass of water can hold much more than meets the eye.

Governmental agencies such as the US Environmental Protection Agency set and regulate maximum levels for dozens of specific contaminants falling under six categories:

- ❑ Microorganisms (primarily bacterial, viral and protozoan).
- ❑ Inorganic Chemicals (largely trace minerals).
- ❑ Organic Chemicals (fumigants, manufacturing by-products).
- ❑ Disinfectants.
- ❑ Disinfection Byproducts.
- ❑ Radionuclides (elements, both natural and manmade, that emit radiation).

Though most public water treatment facilities in North America follow guidelines based on EPA-type levels, research indicates many contaminants, including cancer-producing by-products of the treatment process itself, are often present in treated water. And while governmental standards consider small doses of many contaminants to be safe, there is much disagreement. Some environmental experts consider allowable limits for suspected toxic or cancer-causing pollutants too high. There is also concern about the little explored realm of contaminants' synergistic effect or possible "greater when combined" action on our bodies. So while the tap water in North America is certainly a cleaner source of water than in many places in the world, for an increasing number of consumers, tap water is no longer the drink of the day.

If you are trying to decide between tap water, distilled water, ionized water (i.e. water that has undergone a process to segregate its acid and alkaline content), reverse osmosis filtered water, MRET water (i.e. water with a linear line-up of smaller molecules) or bottled water, remember first of all that almost any clean water is better than not enough water. Water is so important that on one hand, it hardly seems worth quibbling about whether it came from the tap or a filtration system. Once you have ensured your child is having sufficient water intake each day, however, it is worth taking a look at the type of water he is drinking. Quantity is important, but water quality—ensuring your child is drinking clean water—also plays a role in health.

There are enough studies on the long-term impact of chemicals in tap water (i.e. chlorine, pesticides) that practicing some measure of water purification makes sense. Inexpensive systems like a Brita™ filter cannot produce the level of clean water a multi-step process can, but they are a good place to start. As space and finances allow, purchase a home filtration system (i.e. personal favourites are an MRET, British Berkefeld or Santevia™ water system), or move to buying purified bottled water—preferably in refillable glass bottles or plastic bottles numbered 2, 4, 5 as these types of plastic do not leach Bisphenol A, a hormone disrupter.

Water's Importance

The role that water plays in optimal health is sorely misunderstood and underestimated. Quite simply, water is the body's most important nutrient. Dr. Batmanghelidj, in his book *Your Body's Many Cries for Water*, states that water is the medium in which life in our body is expressed. At conception your child was surrounded by water and for his 9 months of pre-birth growth, he was carried in a water-filled amniotic sac.

> ### DIGGING DEEPER
> ### Clean Water
>
> **Want to do a little water research of your own? Try these resources from a well-known water expert: *Your Body's Many Cries for Water; Water: For Health, For Healing, For Life: You're not Sick, You're Thirsty!;* and *Water Cures: Drugs Kill: How Water Cured Incurable Diseases,* all by Dr. Fereydoon Batmanghelidj.**

After birth—though we see very little of it—our body fluids really are everywhere. Between 57-70% of our body weight is made up of water. The different ratios come about because of age and gender. With regard to age, a larger percentage of infants and children's weight is water. With gender, about 65% of men's body weight is water, while women, who generally have a higher proportion of fatty tissue that does not as readily hold water, have a lower percentage of water. Water starts by filling and bathing each of our body's 100 trillion cells. Then it makes up the fluid that travels the 60,000 miles or 100,000 km of veins and arteries in our body. About 98% of intestinal, gastric, saliva and pancreatic juices are water as are 92% of our blood and our tears. Water goes virtually everywhere and surrounds virtually every bit of tissue in our system.

And while clean water has many roles in health, one of the most important is the natural protection it helps provide against a variety of infectious diseases including influenza, pneumonia, whooping cough and measles. The performance of your tissues and their resistance to illness and injury is absolutely dependent on the quality and quantity of water you drink. When the cells are supplied with sufficient pure water, they can fight off viral attack. If body cells are water-starved they become parched, dry and shriveled, making them easy prey for viruses.

How More Water Can Lead to Less Weight

Though it was conducted on adults, rather than *KIB*-aged participants, a recent study on water's impact on weight loss finally confirmed what health experts have suspected. When you drink more water, you lose more weight—and keep that weight off long term.[1] There is yet no clear understanding as to the exact reasons for the "more water-less weight" link, but here are a few possibilities.

Among water's many roles is its task of holding nutritional elements in solution and acting as a transportation medium for those elements. Another transport function, and one of water's most important jobs, is holding body wastes and toxins in solution and carrying them to where they can be removed from the body. If you would like to see your child at a healthy weight, it is critical that he receive essential nutrients and that he rid himself, in a timely manner, of the toxins that are natural by-products of eating, breathing and moving. Sufficient water intake helps that happen.

More water can also lead to less weight when it supports your child's attempts at increasing activity levels: water acts as a lubricant for our joints and soft tissues; water helps maintain normal body temperature by allowing heat to escape as water evaporates from our skin; and water provides the medium for red blood cells to transport oxygen to the tissues.

Most importantly—although with water, importance is rather a relative term—water provides the liquid environment in which enzymes can digest food and convert it to energy. Without that energy, we could not survive.

Our bodies give ample indication of water deprivation including dry, parched skin; headaches; dry and brittle hair; chronic constipation; and burning, irritating urination. Likewise, though it happens more rarely than insufficient water intake, our bodies alert us to water overload as well: muscle cramps, slurred speech, nausea, disorientation and confusion. Most often occurring with athletes engaged in high intensity activity that are losing sodium through prolonged and excessive sweating (i.e. marathons, triathlons), water intoxication is the result of drinking sufficiently high amounts of water to produce a low concentration of sodium in the blood. Be sure your child knows the beginning signs of both insufficient and excessive water intake and help him work toward drinking the right amount of clean water. Depending upon the season and his activity level that means 6-11 glasses [1.5 litres-2.75 litres] each day.

KIB Stories for Life

Again can't thank you enough for all your help! My son Josh is so disciplined! He has really taken ownership and I just thank the Lord daily. This is going to help him his whole life! He is a new man!

Rose

C – Clean Water 101

An Essential Nutrient for Every Body

The metabolism of food requires many nutrients and co-factors; enzymes, hydrochloric acid, bile, minerals and vitamins are all critical components in the correct break down and utilization of nutrients. Water is particularly important. Even mild dehydration will slow metabolism affecting both efficiency of nutrient absorption as well as ability to lose weight. Sufficient water intake also enhances kidney function, which in turn puts less of a load on the liver. That means the liver's fat-burning ability can function more effectively.

Stay Away From Water's Enemies

Water's roles (i.e. transport of nutrients to cells and toxins away from cells) are hampered by a variety of chemicals and foodstuffs. In order to make best use of the water you drink, avoid excess sodium, refined sugar, alcohol and caffeine—found in coffee, caffeinated teas, hot chocolate and many soft drinks—particularly before exercise. Highly processed foods of any type should also be minimized, as ridding the body of the chemicals they contain requires additional water.

Make Drinking Enough Water a Lifelong Goal

Even once your child is in his healthy weight range, drinking sufficient water continues to be an essential step in maintaining wellness. Additionally, as your child's fat cells become smaller, skin tone and tautness can suffer. Drinking sufficient water ensures cells are well hydrated and plump.

How Much is Enough?

Depending upon the season (i.e. temperature and humidity) and activity level (i.e. increased exertion leads to an increased need) have your child drink 6-11 [1.5 litres-2.75 litres] glasses of water per day. Want more specific direction? Try 4 glasses [1 litre] for every 50 pounds of body weight. Realize too that sometimes the body's thirst signals get misread as messages about hunger. If your child thinks he might be hungry, have him try a large glass of water first. Then 15 minutes later, have him evaluate if he is still hungry or if he was just thirsty and is now fine.

Additional Water Intake Suggestions for Athletes

Drink 1 cup [250ml] of water an hour or two before practices and games or sports events and an additional cup [250ml] 20 minutes before the practice or event begins. During exercise, sip about ½ cup [125ml] of water every 15 minutes and when activity is over, slowly drink 2 [500ml] cups of water for every pound of weight loss during exercise. If your child is drinking enough, his urine should be clear or light yellow.

Chapter 9

E– Eat for Health

One of the very nicest things about life is the way we must regularly stop whatever it is we are doing and devote our attention to eating.

Luciano Pavarotti and William Wright
Pavarotti, My Own Story

The last of *KIB*'s seven factors that are key to achieving and maintaining an appropriate weight is a healthy food intake. Because, as Pavarotti describes, we spend repeated amounts of time and attention on food, it will, in many ways, be the focal point of your child's success. After all, what we put in our mouths grows our bodies. By incorporating the following Food Fundamentals and Simple Food Principles into your family's daily meal planning, your child will be off to a great start in encouraging her body to move into a healthy weight range.

Additionally, for those parents and children that learn better with graphic illustration of a point, this chapter introduces *KIB*'s Healthy Living Pyramid. The Healthy Living Pyramid has, as its foundation, *KIB*'s BALANCE approach, but it also clearly illustrates the six food groups that make up the *Kids in Balance* dietary plan. With *KIB*'s Food Fundamentals, Simple Food Principles and the Healthy Living Pyramid firmly in hand, before long, your child will be easily and naturally walking out a dietary plan designed to help her reach long term wellness.

Food Fundamentals

Standing in front of the volume and diversity of material contained in a bookstore's section on Food and Diet is enough to overwhelm even the most nutritionally savvy parent. Because there is such a maze of confusing—and often contradictory—dietary insight available today, *KIB*'s Food Fundamentals were created to act as a grid through which to evaluate information or as a lens to guide your perspective on healthy food choices. The points are easy to explain to your child and, if presented with some of the examples noted below, are concepts that will quickly become second nature to her and the rest of your family members.

1) Eat things that are meant to be eaten.

In other words, eat real food. Age-old guidelines on what foods to eat as well as how to best prepare foods are still important today and, incidentally, have increasing amounts of scientific backing. Because of potential for infestation by parasites or toxicity (i.e. mercury content), the minimization of foods such as pork, ostrich and shellfish continues to be a good health guideline. You may choose to enjoy these foods on occasion, but do not serve them on a regular basis.

Additionally, as much as possible, avoid fake foods such as artificial colors and flavours, and foods loaded with preservatives and other additives. Your body then has an easier time processing real food and has less waste material to eliminate or store after digestion.

Watch out for, and avoid intake of, artificial sweeteners such as Aspartame™ and Splenda® as well. They are not recommended ingredients in a healthy diet and have the potential to both create significant health challenges, and contribute to obesity.[1]

2) Eat foods as close as possible to their original form.

While not suggesting your child munches on freshly dug from the garden, unwashed potatoes and beets, I am, however, recommending she eat foods that have as little processing and contain as few additives as possible. The nice thing is, you do not need to be a nutritionist to figure out why to avoid processed foods or what that term means, especially if your family has viewed the documentary *Supersize Me* and has seen evidence there of what eating a wide variety of foods not very close to their original form can do to your health!

If you have not yet seen the movie or need a refresher course, ask your child, "Which is closer to its original fresh-from-the-garden-state, a baked potato with butter and chives or its pulverized, re-formed, sweetened and hydrogenated cousin the deep-fried potato patty?" Follow that up with a question on whether a crisp, green Granny Smith apple from the fruit bowl or a hot out of the grease, white flour and sugar-laden apple turnover looks more like its orchard-picked ancestor?

Finally, ask your child where Grandma's amazing recipe for The World's Best Apple Crisp with tart, skin-on apples, rolled oats, butter, honey and cinnamon comes in terms of being close to its original form. The right answer is that a bowl of Grandma's apple crisp will fit somewhere in the middle of the extremes of a fresh, Granny Smith apple and a fast food hot apple pie. While not something to eat on a daily basis, once your child is through **Find Your BALANCE**, that apple crisp would be something your family could have once in a while as a deliciously enjoyed Sometimes Food.

The question often arises as to whether eating close to original form means eating organic. Not necessarily. What I suggest *KIB* families aim for is eating foods that have as much of their original nutritional value as possible and that have as little application or addition of chemicals as possible.

Depending upon factors such as family budget, where a family lives and a family's proximity to locally produced foodstuffs, eating foods as close as possible to original form can take on a variety of appearances. Some families may have the budget and market accessibility that allows them to purchase certified organic, locally grown produce and non-medicated meats and dairy products. Other families may need to rely on conventionally grown and raised but minimally processed food stuffs from the grocery store and will, for example, purchase produce that looks freshest and then wash it well before eating. Still other families, in summer months, will be able to supplement conventionally grown foodstuffs with produce from a local farmers' market, Community Supported Agriculture share (CSA) or backyard garden. The goal is to become more aware of what constitutes healthily produced, real food and to include it in the diet as often as possible.

3) Do not become slave to any dietary plan.

One of the factors that has become increasingly clear as contributing to rising obesity rates is the tendency to choose a magic bullet or quick fix approach over discipline, perseverance and lifestyle change. Thus the rush for the latest and greatest but often unsound diet plan and the subsequent nutritional deficiency, calorie deprivation and lack of foundational food information that have only amplified the weight issues families are trying to address. One size fits all dietary plans that advocate extremely low fat intake; intake of altered fats, processed or artificial foods; significant calorie reduction; or no carbohydrates (remember vegetables are carbohydrates so the *KIB* approach is not a no-carb plan) produce nutritional, metabolic and hormonal imbalances that long term, lead to ill health. And it goes without saying, please stay away from strange and fanatical diets as well. Starting a plan that, for example, rotates through one day on water, one day on tuna and one day on grapefruit is just plain silliness.

Fad dieting—a short term, drastic modification and caloric limitation of food intake that is not something you would be able to incorporate into a healthy lifestyle—just does not work. Long term, extreme caloric restriction leads to ill health and can impact your body's ability to handle an appropriate amount of daily food intake. The usual cycle is: excess weight, a fad diet, initial weight loss, an abandoning of the overly restrictive weight loss plan, a return to the usual style of eating, return of weight lost (and often an even increased number of pounds) and then attempts at another calorie-restrictive approach. Rather than tackling the root causes of the obesity problem, fad dieting is simply an easy and effective way to create a yo-yo dieter.

Bringing that concept down to a more personal level, imagine your child's body thinking it has been stranded on a deserted island, without sufficient food. Then imagine the natural effects as her body compensates for a reduced food supply: metabolism slows, the way the body utilizes stored fat is impacted and there is reduction in nutrient intake, particularly nutrients that can be difficult to get in the first place like essential omega-3 oils or amino acids. Not a great game plan.

Even if you have discovered the healthiest way to eat known to mankind, it still needs to be something that gives you the freedom to have an enjoyable holiday celebration or a family games night with snacks without feeling deprived or alienated.

Simple Food Principles

Once you and your child have a good understanding of the Food Fundamentals, it is time to add a few Simple Food Principles.

1) Minimize refined foods like white flour and sugars.

The word refined sounds like such an elegant word, one that could, in fact, be descriptive of foods to **include** in a healthy diet. Instead, in food industry terms, the refining process is a series of steps that strip nutrients from natural foods and leave them as foodstuffs best to avoid. Whereas the bulk of a family's dietary intake was once grown or hunted locally and eaten in a whole food (i.e. unprocessed, non-medicated) form, with advances in knowledge and expertise—the milling process for example—long-term storage of food became a reality. In flour mills, new equipment meant millers were able to remove the outer, more easily spoiled components of grain—the germ and bran. Now the flour had a longer shelf life and millers were able to store, transport and sell it to a broader market. Their new product, white flour, was less nutritious than its whole grain forerunner, but it had several important factors going for it. Because it was new and less common, it was seen as somewhat of a status symbol and because of its longer shelf life, with increased technology and factory-produced foods, it became the industry standard for use in those processed foods.

Consumption of refined grains and sugars contributes to a loss of essential nutrients, which in turn leads to a variety of other ailments including obesity and digestive disorders. Short term, refined sugar use can cause fatigue, weight gain, arthritis and depression. Long term, the list of potential ailments includes dental cavities, heart disease, yeast overgrowth, hypertension, hypoglycemia and emotional illness. Moving these less than helpful foods out of your family's daily diet and relegating them to a rare Sometimes Foods appearance is one of the best things you can do to help your child reach and maintain health and wellness.

2) Eat enough good quality protein-rich food.

Upon completion of an initial *Food/Mood/Activity Log*, most *KIB* parents discover their child is eating too many carbohydrate-rich foods (i.e. grains, cereals, breads, pastas, crackers, sugars, potatoes, rice and even fruit) in proportion to protein-rich foods (i.e. red meat, chicken, lamb, turkey, fish, legumes, nuts, seeds, eggs, cheese). Even most food charts place a major emphasis on eating large amounts of grain-based foodstuffs at the expense of sufficient recommendation for protein foodstuffs, particularly for those with a Protein Body Type.

Often a simple way to help your child with the transition from too many grains is by addressing snack time food options. Rather than suggesting corn chips and salsa or crackers for a mid-afternoon snack break, provide trail mix and baby carrots or a turkey pepperoni stick and red pepper strips. Next, make sure your child is starting her morning with a yogurt smoothie or an egg or nut butter on sprouted whole grain toast.

Even for children that are very physically active, perhaps training for a cross-country event or swim meet, fuelling up on carbohydrates or "carb loading" is not generally recommended. A modest amount of a carbohydrate-rich food (i.e. fruit, starchy vegetable, slice of sprouted grain bread) can be very helpful, especially for body types that do better on higher amounts of carbohydrate-rich foods, but it needs to be coupled with small but regular amounts of protein-rich foods.

3) Get enough healthy fat.

"Wait a minute," you might say; "I thought the *KIB* approach would have our family cutting fat from our diet." And in some ways you are right. All the unnatural, altered, chemically-processed fats like the trans fats found in many French fries, chips, donuts, snack foods, salad dressings and crackers should be minimized or eliminated. They are simply not in the right form to be useful to the body and, much like trying to put a square peg in a round hole, create havoc as the body tries to make do with them.

Fats and fat-rich foods that have been used for generations, and that have been shown to be necessary and of great benefit, however, should be taken on a daily basis. That means including foods like butter, extra virgin olive oil, coconut oil, fish oils, nuts, seeds and avocados in your diet.

4) Watch the dairy intake.

The *KIB* approach allows for modest amounts of dairy products as part of your child's daily protein-rich food intake. Medium fat cheeses and yogurt are decent protein sources for many people and can play a part in a healthy diet. If your child tolerates dairy well, have them eat dairy products in moderation, but, if possible, look for organic, and if available where you live, even raw sources. If your child has allergies or intolerances to dairy products, keep them out of her diet and omit dairy products in *KIB* Recipes or make recommended substitutions.

5) Increase your vegetable intake, and have a bit of fruit.

Fresh fruits and vegetables are valuable sources of a variety of vitamins, minerals and enzymes and, as well, contain a variety of phytochemicals that play an important role in disease prevention and eradication. In their antioxidant role, the body uses fruits and vegetables to neutralize the damage caused by free radicals, enemies of good health that are produced by stress, toxins and natural body processes. Current research also seems to indicate that certain plant food properties help properly regulate the body's blood vessel growth, ensuring that fat cells do not become too well fed and thus grow more rapidly than they should.

Fresh produce also contains high water content, a variety of valuable fibres, and enzymes—catalysts for many of the body's chemical processes. Vegetables should be consumed daily, both raw and cooked, in relatively high amounts (i.e. 5-7 servings/day or even more if your child enjoys vegetables).

Where does fruit intake factor into the *KIB* plan? Depending upon body type and *KIB* dietary phase, 0-3 servings of fruit can also be eaten each day. As much as possible, choose whole fruit rather than fruit juice. The additional fibre contained in whole fruits contributes in a variety of ways to good health, including slowing the metabolism of the fructose naturally contained in fruit.

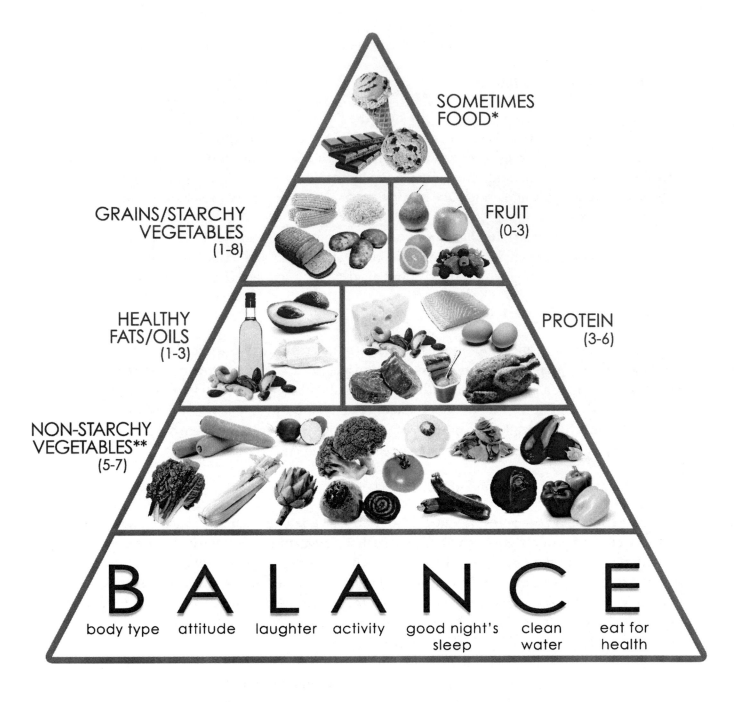

SOMETIMES FOOD*

GRAINS/STARCHY VEGETABLES (1-8)

FRUIT (0-3)

HEALTHY FATS/OILS (1-3)

PROTEIN (3-6)

NON-STARCHY VEGETABLES** (5-7)

BALANCE

body type   attitude   laughter   activity   good night's sleep   clean water   eat for health

* Eat sparingly
  - sugary drinks & foods
  - refined grains, breads pastas, white rice
  - alcohol

** Choose a range of colours and a variety of textures

Figure 2. Healthy Living Pyramid

KIB's Healthy Living Pyramid

Since the late 1800s we have seen creation of North American governmental publications on dietary recommendations. Over the past number of decades, in both Canada and the United States, however, there have been a variety of modifications made as to the number of food groups, the recommended number of servings, and the types of foods included in the recommendations. While there are helpful suggestions in these types of dietary recommendations, *KIB* has formulated a Healthy Living Pyramid that realigns some of the food groups by type and priority. By including all BALANCE components, this pyramid presents a more complete picture in addressing the wide range of factors that facilitate your child reaching a healthy weight and optimal wellness.

Changes from more conventional food recommendations include the fact the Healthy Living Pyramid differentiates between fruits and vegetables. Both are healthy foods, but because of fruit's natural higher sugar content, it is a food group needed in different amounts by different body types. The Healthy Living Pyramid also includes a wide daily-recommended serving range for protein-rich foods as well as for grains/starchy vegetables and fruit. This allows for emphasis on different food groups for different body types (i.e. proteins such as red meats for the Protein Body Type whose fuel mix optimally includes a higher percentage of purine-rich foods—a specific category of protein foods that are a helpful source of energy for Protein Body Types).

Finally, the Healthy Living Pyramid recognizes increasing research showing the emotional and physical health consequences of widely fluctuating blood sugar/insulin levels,[2] and, the impact of different types of foodstuffs on blood sugar levels.[3,4] Therefore, instead of recommending an across the board amount of grains and fruit, *KIB* provides opportunity for the dietary individuation required by different body types to keep blood sugar levels stable. This means lower amounts of fruits, starchy vegetables and grains for Protein Body Types, higher amounts of those foodstuffs for Carbohydrate Body Types and a moderate amount of fruits and grains for Mixed Body Types.

Protein (3-6 servings of protein-rich food a day)

Next to water, protein is the most abundant nutrient in our bodies. We require protein to develop and maintain muscle, bone, vital organs, blood, hair, nails and other body tissue. As well, in order to produce hormones, enzymes, antibodies and blood cells, our bodies need a regular intake of this important nutrient. Protein is also an essential factor in the development of a healthy immune system. Without adequate supplies of appropriate protein, we are less able to fight off infection and we recover more slowly from illness when it strikes.

During digestion, protein is broken down into protein building blocks called amino acids. Our bodies can make eleven of the twenty known amino acids we use to form and repair various organs and tissues. The other nine amino acids are generally regarded as essential as they need to be supplied through diet. In order to maintain our health, a good variety of protein-rich foods should be regularly consumed.

Very occasionally, if amino acid deficiency is considerable (i.e. mood imbalances and cravings are not reduced by following *KIB* principles and your child's doctor has ruled out other possible causes for the moods and cravings), and is unable to be met with dietary protein intake alone, supplementation of individual amino acids may be required. See *KIB-Friendly Supplements* (p. 196) for information and meet with your health care professional for information on correct type and dosage of amino acids.

Foods that are included in the protein-rich group include meat (i.e. beef, bison, lamb, pork, elk, venison, moose, rabbit); fish (i.e. anchovies, bluefish, flounder, halibut, Pacific cod, prawns, scallops, sole, wild salmon); poultry (i.e. chicken, turkey, Cornish game hen, duck); legumes (i.e. split peas, snap peas, snow peas, chickpeas, lentils and beans—pinto, Romano, black, white, kidney); nuts (i.e. almonds, cashews, filberts, pecans, peanuts, walnuts, pine nuts, Brazil nuts, macadamia nuts, nut butters); seeds (i.e. flax, sesame, hemp, sunflower, chia, salba, seed butters); dairy products (i.e. cheese, yogurt, kefir, sour cream, milk); and eggs.

Protein Body Types require a higher percentage of protein-rich foods in their daily fuel mix. For optimum mood or physical and mental energy they usually need to include, on a regular basis, at least small amounts of what are called the medium or higher purine-rich proteins found in red meats, darker poultry (i.e. game birds or thighs and drumsticks of chicken and turkey) and richer seafood such as anchovies, sardines, herring and salmon.

Carbohydrate Body Types require less protein-rich foods in their daily fuel mix and usually need more of it in a lower purine-rich form such as legumes, nuts and seeds. They often see a negative impact on mood, energy or mental clarity with intake of the higher purine-rich foods.

Mixed Body Types usually do best on a combination of higher and lower purine-rich foods. They need to experiment with the exact fuel mix to see what best suits their individual body type.

Fats (1-3 servings a day)

Among other functions, fats are used by the body to build cell walls, help with pain and inflammation, grow healthy hair, skin and nails, and work to produce and balance hormones—a very good thing for everyone but particularly for children and adolescents. There are healthy fats, some of which are essential fats that the body cannot make and need to be supplied through diet, and unhealthy fats that should, as much as possible, be avoided.

Healthy Fats—Healthy fats are supplied by nuts, seeds, avocadoes and oils such as extra virgin olive oil, virgin olive oil, coconut oil, butter, sesame oil, grapeseed oil, walnut oil, sunflower oil, hemp oil and flaxseed oil. They are also found in oily fish such as salmon, halibut, herring, cod, sardines and mackerel. Most oils should not be heated as cooking destroys the essential fatty acids or encourages rancidity. Coconut oil, a long-used saturated fat, is an exception to the "no heat" rule and is the best choice for cooking, particularly higher heat cooking. Coconut oil also works well for lightly sautéing foods or baking, although butter and grapeseed oil can occasionally be used at lower heats as well. Less heat-resistant oils (i.e. extra virgin olive oil, walnut oil) should be used to drizzle over cooked vegetables or in salad dressings.

Essential Fats—Also part of the healthy fat category, Essential Fatty Acids (EFAs) are fats that are as essential as vitamins and minerals for optimum health and, as the body cannot create them, need to be supplied on a daily basis through diet or supplement. Unlike other healthy fats that play a large role in energy production, EFAs are used mainly for hormonal, structural and nerve functions, and are found predominantly in oily fish and some nuts and seeds. We need an intake of both linoleic acid (LA), an omega-6 fatty acid found in safflower oil, sunflower oil, poppy seeds, hemp seeds, sesame seeds and wheat germ, as well as alpha linolenic acid (ALA), an omega-3 fatty acid found in fish and fish oils, flaxseeds, pumpkin seeds, chia seeds, kiwi and walnuts.

Unhealthy Fats—Altered fats (i.e. fats that have been negatively impacted by heating or hydrogenation) or fats found in meats with an unhealthy ratio of saturated fat that results when animals are fed an abundance of grains rather than grass-fed, fall into the category of unhealthy fats. Realize that even good EFAs can become unhealthy if heated or altered. Watch both the type of oil you are purchasing as well as how it is processed (i.e. look for as natural, unrefined and cold-pressed a source as possible). Store oils in dark containers, away from heat and light.

Carbohydrates

Along with protein and fat, carbohydrates are one of the three macronutrients our bodies need for optimum health. In the *KIB* program, the carbohydrate-rich food group is divided into three sub-categories: grains, vegetables and fruit. Because they are derived from plant sources, good quality carbohydrate-rich foods are usually naturally low in fat and cholesterol. Once carbohydrate foodstuffs are processed, however, many of their valuable nutrients are removed or destroyed and their natural goodness is often altered with sugars, unhealthy fats or chemicals (i.e. as happens with French fries, croissants, pastries, some crackers and muffins, and fried snacks such as doughnuts and most chips).

While everyone benefits from an intake of carbohydrate-rich foods, depending upon body type, there needs to be a monitoring of the type and amount of carbohydrates eaten each day. Every body type needs carbohydrates from vegetables, but Protein, Carbohydrate and Mixed Body Types need starchy vegetables, grain and fruit-source carbohydrates in differing types and amounts.

In order to achieve and maintain wellness, Protein Body Types often need to limit their starchy vegetable/grain intake to 1-2 servings/day and keep their fruit intake to 1-2 servings/day. Carbohydrate Body Types do better on a higher percentage of both grains and fruit, and Mixed Body Types will need an amount that falls somewhere in between the amount that keeps a Protein and Carbohydrate Body Type functioning optimally. In order to best help your child reach and maintain a healthy weight, it is important to complete *KIB*'s *Body Type Survey*, and understand the information in the Body Type chapter and in *KIB*'s *Fuel Mix Guidelines* so you know what varieties and amount of carbohydrate-rich foods best fit in your child's optimum fuel mix.

Vegetables (5-7 servings a day)—In order to help provide the vitamins, minerals, fibre and enzymes your child needs to maintain optimal health, she needs to eat a minimum of five servings of lower glycemic vegetables—non-starchy varieties with a slower rate of digestion and absorption—each day. Vegetables are versatile and flavourful, and can be served in a variety of ways, including in recipes that, believe it or not, can become real family favourites.

As with many things you will pass on to your child, your admonitions to "Eat your veggies!" rank right near the top for wise words of counsel. On a regular basis, researchers are discovering more and more phytochemicals and, in turn, finding more ways these plant compounds work to protect health and prevent disease, including preventing obesity.

While all natural plant-sourced foods contain phytochemicals, beans, fruits, herbs and particularly vegetables, contain high amounts of a wide variety of phytochemicals. Increasing your family's vegetable intake means gaining a wide variety of healthful benefits.

Grains/Starchy Vegetables (1-8 servings a day)— Regardless of body type, when grains are in the fuel mix, minimize or eliminate white flour-based products and make use of whole grains. Realize, though, that occasionally people have trouble tolerating even natural whole grains. For some it is an issue with gluten—the protein in many grains, particularly barley, rye, oats and wheat. For others it may be because certain grain components (i.e. phytic acid) interfere with digestion and mineral absorption. In these instances it can be best to use non-gluten grains (i.e. quinoa, rice) and starchy vegetables (i.e. sweet potato, potatoes, beets) as primary carbohydrate-rich food sources; and, in order to reduce phytic acid and increase nutritional content and digestibility, ensure that grains are sprouted before serving (i.e. sprouted grain breads).

Fruit (0-3 servings/day)—Fruit is a source of vitamins and minerals, antioxidants, and fibre. While fruit can make an excellent snack, particularly for Carbohydrate and Mixed Body Types or when paired with nutrient dense protein-rich food such as nuts or a piece of cheese, for Protein Body Types, it is important to monitor the amount of fruit intake. Most fruits are high in natural sugars and therefore will be used sparingly by Protein Body Types and for all body types during *KIB*'s **Find Your BALANCE.**

Fruit juices can have a small part to play (i.e. ½ cup/125ml per day) in a healthy diet for some body types as well. Generally, however, if your child is thirsty, make water her usual beverage of choice and ensure virtually all fruit servings are a whole piece of fruit rather than fruit juice.

Snacks (2-3 servings a day)

While snacks do not constitute a separate *KIB* food group, they are a vitally important part of the *KIB* program and a welcome aspect of most children's—and many adults'—day. Why the suggestion of 3 meals and 2-3 snacks (or 5-6 mini-meals) per day?

- ❑ Because of relative stomach size, many children are able to sustain better-balanced blood sugar levels and, therefore, better balanced energy throughout the day.
- ❑ Balanced blood sugar levels (and the avoidance of "eat ASAP" messages) mean your child is able to make better choices about types of food to eat and how much food to consume.

There are two primary reasons for widely fluctuating blood sugar levels. First blood sugar levels take a significant drop when your child waits too long between meals or snacks. The second, and more complex reason begins with the large blood sugar level increases that occur after eating refined grains and sugars. Those increases alert the pancreas to secrete significant amounts of insulin, but once insulin has done its job of shuttling the excess glucose that is produced from that type of snack to cells for storage, the result is a drop in blood sugar levels. Either way—too long a wait between eating or refined grain and sugar intake—there can be triggered a set of insulin and blood sugar level fluctuations that ultimately result in low blood sugar levels. In turn, because the body then knows it needs to increase blood sugar levels again, there is a critical hunger message sent to the brain, and the need to be fed becomes urgent.

KIB's snack suggestions are designed to help your child avoid widely fluctuating blood sugar levels in two ways: the timing of snacks and the type of snack. When your child has a regular intake of food, and when that food contains both a nutritionally dense food source (i.e. protein and fat), and fibrous voluminous food (i.e. raw vegetables), she will feel a sense of Comfortable Fullness and avoid hunger. It will be much easier for your child to make healthy food choices and to eat appropriate amounts of food, a major support in helping your child reach her health goals.

Snacks should generally consist of a small portion of protein-rich food (i.e. about 2 ounces or ½ the size of a deck of cards) and a small serving of vegetables or occasionally a small portion of protein-rich food and a small fruit. The portions may look small but remember that these foods are the types that enable your child to feel full for longer. A few options are given in the Top *KIB* Snack Suggestions chart below, but get creative on your own as well.

As your child progresses into **Build Your BALANCE**, she will also be able to occasionally add in small portions of Sometimes Foods (not recommended until having completed 4 weeks of **Build Your BALANCE**). While a little more fun or celebratory, these foods should be eaten in moderation (i.e. 3 times/week and in controlled portions; reduce if adverse reactions occur).

Top *KIB* Snack Suggestions

Protein and Veggie or Fruit	Protein and Veggie or Fruit	Sometimes Snacks
1 cheese string 5-6 baby carrots	1 tablespoon almond butter 2 stalks celery	1 ounce [25g] dark chocolate 10 almonds
1 turkey pepperoni stick ½ red pepper	1 chicken kabob and tzatziki (5-½ inch [1 cm] cubes meat and 1 cup [100g] veggies)	½ cup [90g] **Trail Mix** with 15 chocolate chips
½ cup [125ml] **Hummus** 10 cucumber slices	1 serving of **No-dough Pizza** with vegetables	½ cup [125ml] homemade pudding
2 small beef deli slices 2 large leaves romaine lettuce	1 tablespoon sunflower seeds ½ grapefruit	½ cup [125ml] good quality ice cream or gelato
1 hard boiled egg ½ yellow pepper	⅓ cup [75g] cottage cheese 1 cup [200g] cantaloupe	1 cup [25g] corn chips with salsa 1 inch [2 cm] cube Jarlsberg
¼ cup [60ml] **Ranch Dressing** 1 cup [100g] raw vegetables	1 inch [2 cm] cube Gouda 6 strawberries	1 cup [10g] popcorn sprinkled with 1 tablespoon Parmesan cheese
1 inch [2 cm] cube Gouda 2 medium onion slices	½ cup [90g] **Trail Mix** (dried nuts and lightly sweetened cranberries)	1 small protein-rich homemade granola bar
1 tablespoon cream cheese 5-6 snap peas	10 pecans 1 small mandarin orange	1 small protein-rich homemade cookie
1 tablespoon cream cheese baked on ½ red pepper	1 tablespoon peanut butter 1 small apple, sliced	smoothie (½ cup [125ml] each yogurt, blueberries & banana)
10 almonds 5-6 carrot sticks	1 inch [2 cm] cube cheddar 10 green grapes	1 cup [25g] potato chips (pota- toes, oil, salt) and 1 cheese string

Fibre

Most people do not eat enough fibre, getting on average 15 grams each day. For digestive health, for proper functioning of the colon and to provide a food source for the good bacteria that help keep us healthy, intake should average 25-30 grams of fibre per day. To put that in perspective and help you understand what you will need to add to the menu to up your family's fibre intake, note that most fruits, vegetables and whole grains have at least 2-4 grams of fibre per serving. Whole grains such as brown rice and barley; vegetables like sweet potatoes, snow peas and baked potatoes, with skin; and apples and pear, with skin, are a high source of fibre with 4-6 grams of fibre per servings. Cooked legumes; most nuts and seeds; berries; and dried fruit, are a very high source of fibre with more than 6 grams of fibre per serving.

One of Your Body's Best Friends—Unlike refined sugars which, when not used for energy, can very quickly be stored as your body's fat reserves, fibre is largely indigestible and provides a sense of fullness and satisfaction. An added bonus is that fibre also helps slow down the absorption of sugar into our system. For instance, among other benefits, it is the presence of fibre in fruit that makes eating a piece of whole fruit a much better choice than drinking fruit juice. Finally, fibre cleans up. Fibre is able to push waste matter out of the body as it makes its way through the digestive tract. An appropriately speedy transit time—time between food intake and food elimination—is important for optimal health.

Boosting Fibre Intake—The key to upping fibre intake is to gradually increase the amount of fibre-rich foods you eat to give your body a chance to get used to the change. Too much too soon can cause bloating, gas and feelings of discomfort. Here are a few other tips:

- Drink plenty of water. It helps your body use fibre properly.
- Choose carbohydrate-rich foods such as sprouted grain breads, starchy vegetables, basmati and wild rice, and quinoa instead of processed and refined grains.
- Enjoy a wide variety and amount of vegetables and a wide variety and select amount of fruits, with the skins whenever possible.
- Include fibre-filled legumes such as chickpeas, navy beans and lentils in your meals.
- Snack on fibre-rich foods such as carrots, snap peas, nuts and seeds, and body type-appropriate amounts of apples, berries and starchy vegetables. Eat a variety of plant foods. This ensures you get a full complement of the different types of fibre and nutrients.

KIB Stories for Life

Rheana is doing very well. As for the actual weight loss we haven't weighed her lately. She looks healthy, is getting taller and some people have said she looks great! The absolutely BEST result from KIB is her knowledge of food and portions!!! Never would she have learned this at such a critical age had we not been part of the program. She is so aware of what is healthy and what's not! She certainly has many times where her choices could be better BUT she is aware of her decisions. We both thank you for your support!!

Bonnie

E – Eat for Health Summary

Cut Way Back on Sugar and Refined Grains

In the short term, consumption of refined sugar/grains can contribute to fatigue, weight gain, arthritis and depression. Over the long term, the list of potential ailments includes: dental cavities, heart disease, yeast overgrowth, hypertension, hypoglycemia, high cholesterol and emotional illness. Whole grains play a supporting role in the *KIB* plan but depending upon body type, should be used in limited amounts, particularly with body types that do best on higher protein-rich food intake and starches in the form of root vegetables.

Eat Appropriate Amounts of Meat

Most North Americans are of the body type that achieves better health with the inclusion of at least small amounts of animal products in their diet. Including meats like beef, poultry, bison, lamb, fish and wild game in your family's food intake provides a variety of beneficial nutrients including protein, certain B vitamins and iron. For Carbohydrate Body Types, ensure you get a sufficient intake of protein from vegetable sources such as nuts, seeds and legumes or the occasional egg, lighter meat or fish.

Maximize Your Vegetable Intake and Eat a Fruit or Two or Three a Day

Vegetables and fruit are great sources of a variety of vitamins, minerals and enzymes—catalysts for many of the body's chemical processes. They also contain a wealth of phyto—the Greek work for plant—chemicals that play an important role in disease prevention and eradication, and healthy weight maintenance. Include frequent and plentiful servings of raw and cooked vegetables each day (i.e. 5-7 servings or even more if your child enjoys vegetables) and, depending upon body type, 1-3 fruits per day.

Be Wise with Dairy Intake

A cheese string or scoop of cottage cheese—optimally organic—paired with a handful of raw vegetables can be a good snack, especially for a Protein Body Type. While many children can include 1-2 daily servings of dairy as part of their protein-rich food intake, if your child has trouble tolerating dairy products, eliminate them. Instead include a wide variety of other protein-rich food sources along with calcium-rich foods such as greens, sesame seeds, white beans, almonds and sardines.

Get Enough Healthy Fat

Fats provide the most concentrated source of energy for the body, are essential for the manufacturing of cells, aid in calcium absorption and carry fat-soluble vitamins. Avoid processed, hydrogenated and trans fats, and instead use mainly fat-rich foodstuffs that have a long tradition of supporting health—healthy meats and dairy as well as olive oil, butter, coconut oil, nuts, seeds and avocadoes.

Chapter 10

Getting Started

It's a job that's never started that takes the longest to finish.

J. R. R. Tolkien

The *Kids in Balance* plan is a unique, multi-phased—**Find**, **Build** and **Keep Your BALANCE** phases—and multi-faceted—B-A-L-A-N-C-E—lifestyle approach to healthy weight achievement and maintenance. And though it will require time and effort for you and your child to implement, if properly prepared for, it is an easy and positively effective way to do life.

The Need to Prepare

Human nature is often quick acting and impulsive. We see the latest, greatest gadget, diet, exercise equipment, computer software, or toy and clothing trend and have to have it—and have to have it now. While this may work in your family's favour when shopping for amazing deals on travel vacations or catching a glimpse of the last of a farmer's batch of freshly picked blueberries, it is not a good way to begin the *Kids in Balance* program.

Tackling lifestyle change requires preparation so there is sufficient understanding of what lies ahead, as well as to ensure the plans, supplies and motivation are firmly in place before beginning the journey. You and your child have a much higher chance of health and wellness success if you carefully study this book (and if you choose, the bonus accompanying online support materials at www.kidsinbalance.net), take the time to complete the steps and activities outlined in these resources, and walk the *Kids in Balance* program through in the way it is designed.

What to Expect

Before you begin *KIB*'s first phase, **Find Your BALANCE**, you will need a week of preparation time. These seven days are about maintaining status quo in the areas of food intake, physical activity and screen time, and keeping a record of those activities as you learn more about the *KIB* approach. After your week of preparation, you and your child will begin the three-week phase, **Find Your BALANCE**. During the first week of **Find Your BALANCE** you will gradually introduce a few small dietary and lifestyle changes. The last two weeks of **Find Your BALANCE** consist of a gentle, food-based, cleanse. This part of the phase includes a very specific dietary plan of natural foods that includes vegetables, protein-rich foods and fats but eliminates sugars, grains, fruits and starchy vegetables. Among other healthful benefits, this temporary dietary shift allows the body to reduce any potential dependencies on refined sugars and grains, restores a more balanced fluctuation in blood sugar levels and supplies essential nutrients for proper cellular function.

Experience has shown that *KIB* families who prepare well for **Find Your BALANCE** can tackle pretty much any of the dietary and lifestyle challenges life throws at them during *KIB*'s two subsequent phases, **Build Your BALANCE** and **Keep Your BALANCE**, and beyond.

How to Prepare

Both the week of preparation for **Find Your BALANCE**, as well as the three weeks of **Find Your BALANCE** phase, have their own helpful *Day-at-a-Glance Guidelines* (p. 223) with tips on how to cover all of *KIB*'s BALANCE factors on a daily basis. The guidelines help to keep things easy and on track, and will be an important key to your child's success. Looking at the preparation for **Find Your BALANCE** with a broader view than do the *Day-at-a-Glance Guidelines*, however, there are four simple steps to getting ready for **Find Your BALANCE**. Once those are read and understood, you are ready to begin!

1) Start prepping attitude and emotions.

During your preparation week for **Find Your BALANCE**, you will have tasks to complete that encompass many factors in successful weight loss. For this week, however, you **do NOT modify your normal dietary/lifestyle routines**. Your family's emotional preparation will include completing a *Food, Mood, Activity Log* (looking at the link between food choices and emotions); determining your child's motivators (see *Finding Your Motivators*, p. 213); and establishing short and long-term goals (see *Setting Your Goals*, p. 214).

When helping your child work through the *Finding Your Motivators* worksheet, ask questions and get clarity on the types of motivators that make sense for and encourage your child. Make use of rewards that are more material in nature and that may incur some degree of financial cost (i.e. a public swim pass, clothing items or cash toward a more costly item or event), as well as rewards that have no financial cost but are likely as equally important to your child (i.e. increased privileges, opportunity to choose the weekly family night game or an excused chore).

Avoid using poor quality Sometimes Foods (i.e. junk foods) as motivators. While the occasional healthy-ingredient chocolate chip cookie or bag of baked, chemical-free chips might make it on the motivator list, it does not make sense to primarily reward your child with things that are not good for him and that have likely contributed to his being in his current overweight situation. Instead affirm positive behaviour, reward goal attainment or celebrate special occasions with one-on-one parent time, special outdoor activities (i.e. a trip to the zoo or water slides) or non-food gifts such as a Frisbee or indoor activity supplies (i.e. model car kit, craft material, kite-making supplies).

Additional tips you will want to explore to help prepare family attitudes and emotions include suggestions for dealing with stress (see chapter 5 - Laughter and Play) and fitting a healthy nutritional plan into your budget (see *KIB on a Budget*, p. 199).

In order to help you and your child easily keep track of your consistency in handling all the BALANCE factors during *KIB*'s 3-Phase Program, you will also need to photocopy the *KIB How Am I Doing? Chart* (p. 221) or download the chart at www.kidsinbalance.net/kib-resources-1.html. Have it handy to post on the fridge or a bulletin board so the chart can be completed each day of **Find Your BALANCE** and periodically throughout **Build** and **Keep Your BALANCE** phases. Either print enough copies to have one for each day or insert a copy inside a plastic protector page. That way the daily checkmarks can be made on the protector page with a washable felt pen, markings wiped off each morning and the page re-used.

2) Begin re-organizing your kitchen and chore list.

Tasks to do with the physical aspects of achieving a healthier weight are also required during your week of preparation. These tasks focus on going over *KIB* material to learn more about healthier eating and functional fitness. By the end of your preparation week you will understand the need for the gradual reduction of refined grain, sugar and caffeine intake. Likewise you will understand why you will shortly be increasing intake of water, healthy protein-rich foods and vegetables. You will find lots of helpful nutrition information in chapter 9 - Eat for Health (make special note of *KIB*'s Healthy Living Pyramid) as well as support for clearing out less-than-healthful food choices in the *Kitchen Substitutes, Natural Sweeteners* and *Healthy Foods List* in Appendix 7.

3) Get on with the paperwork.

Some of the homework you and your child will do in the preparation week before you begin **Find Your BALANCE** includes recording body type as well as baseline diet, measurements and activity levels. Work with your child to complete the *KIB Body Type Survey* (p. 179) per instructions. The information will be helpful in determining your child's food choices in **Find Your BALANCE** as well as his ideal Fuel Mix through **Build** and **Keep Your BALANCE** phases too.

For your preparation week record your child's food intake, moods and physical activity in the *Food/Mood/Activity Log*. That first week's record will be your child's normal pattern of eating and activity. As well, in the activity column, please record your child's sleep patterns and daily amount of screen time—the amount of time your child spends in front of the television, computer or playing video games and texting. **Please do not modify your child's normal dietary/lifestyle routines for your week of preparation.** This will help you determine where challenges may be and suggests the best *KIB* tools to help with those challenges.

At some point during your preparation week, make a note of your child's baseline weight, height and measurements on *KIB*'s *Measure-up Chart* (p. 212) and, if using a skinfold caliper, note body fat ratio per Taking Healthy Measurements instructions (p. 77). Also take several photos of your child. Although this can be a challenging time of recognizing a difficult reality, it is important to take the measurements and photos with your child both to ensure accuracy in recording his starting place and to be supportive and encouraging. Re-do weight and measurements every two weeks, with particular emphasis on measurements rather than weight; lean tissue is denser than fat tissue and with increased activity levels comes increased lean tissue that may result in minimal or non-existent scale movement some weeks.

4) Prepare for gradual dietary change in the first week of Find Your BALANCE.

Once you complete your week of preparation, it is time to move into the three weeks of **Find Your BALANCE**. Therefore during your preparation week, not only will you do kitchen organization, it is also important to give thought to the gradual modifications in diet and exercise that are a part of the first week of **Find Your BALANCE**. Take a look ahead at the appropriate *Day-at-a-Glance Guidelines* for suggestions as to how to slowly incorporate change. Then stock the pantry with the types of snacks and meal items that will make that transition week go well.

Food Logs: Why *KIB* Loves Them

Though at times, completing a daily food intake form and noting corresponding moods and activity may feel like a bit of a make work project, I recommend the use of *Food/Mood/Activity Logs* for several very important reasons.

Food/Mood/Activity Logs Help with Accuracy—It is easy to miscalculate important details on food intake if one tries to use recall alone. No one's memory is failsafe and you or your child may forget about a quickly grabbed snack, underestimate the amount of food eaten or be unclear as to exactly when a food was consumed. Food logs help you and your child keep a more accurate recording of the types, volume and timing of foods eaten each day. If you are away from the house for the day, take the *Food/Mood/Activity Log* with you; jot food intake down on a scrap of paper to transfer to the log later; or text yourself a list of your child's food intake so as not to forget.

Food/Mood/Activity Logs Help with Understanding—When food intake is recorded along with activity and mood, it is easier for you and your child to see the correlation between food intake and emotion; food intake and desire for physical activity; or food intake under certain social or environmental circumstances. The correlation between amount of food intake (i.e. energy intake) and amount of exercise (i.e. energy expenditure) and your child's ability to reduce excess fat in light of that ratio is also more clearly seen. You may find that white bread or pasta intake contributes to tummy bloating, excess refined sugar depresses your child's moods or insufficient intake of protein-rich foods triggers a quick return of hunger. Additionally you may discover that certain situations (i.e. family movie night, nervousness about an exam) trigger eating of certain foods or overeating in general. When *Food/Mood/Activity Logs* are kept, your child can see the impact of food choices on a wide range of physical and emotional levels (i.e. bloating, physical lethargy, lack of mental clarity, moodiness).

Food/Mood/Activity Logs Help with Accountability—When you and your child have made the commitment to move toward a healthier lifestyle or set goals as to the types of foods you want to begin to eat more regularly, *Food/Mood/Activity Logs* help determine if those goals are being reached. When there is an accurate recording of the volume and types of foods eaten in a day, your child has begun to own the fact that what he puts in his mouth grows his body. It then becomes far more difficult to live in denial about the quantity or quality of the foods being eaten. Even more importantly, with the recording of food intake, activity and moods, your child will begin to see the direct correlation between the types and amounts of food eaten, and the fairly immediate responses such as dips or elevations in mood and energy. He will also see emerging patterns of key health factors such as timing of food intake and emotional responses like irritation or anxiety. These are important points in understanding the way wide fluctuations in blood sugar levels or insufficient levels of fullness and sense of satisfaction after eating can contribute to your child's excess weight. That in turn, can be a key point in your child taking responsibility for his choices.

Food/Mood/Activity Logs Help with Lifestyle Change—Because *KIB* promotes making long term changes in a broad range of areas rather than a one-shot or magic bullet approach to health and wellness, *Food/Mood/Activity Logs* can help families see the benefits of a lifetime of eating for:

❑ Blood sugar stabilization.
❑ Sense of satisfaction.

☐ Comfortable Fullness.

☐ Consistent energy.

Fulfilling these four aspects of food intake helps greatly with you and your child's ability to make healthy change last for a lifetime.

Completing a *Food/Mood/Activity Log*

Using a blank copy of *KIB's Food/Mood/Activity Log* or keeping a similar record on the family calendar, record the exact type and amount of food eaten (i.e. 1 granola bar, 2 scrambled eggs in a ½ tsp. of butter, 1 cup beef spaghetti sauce over 2 cups cooked pasta, a 4 ounce candy bar, 10 baby carrots) at all meals and snacks. Be sure to record any beverages consumed as well. Additionally, in the spaces provided, note moods before eating and then again an hour or two after eating. Any activity should be noted as well, including sleep pattern, physical activity or screen time (i.e. 8 hours of restless sleep, 10 minute walk to school, 2 hours of TV, a 1 hour soccer practise, ½ hour of computer). Be precise and honest—no need to "pad" the log with vegetables or physical activity that simply is not happening. *Food/Mood/Activity Log* details provide valuable clues to some of the reasons your child is carrying excess weight, but the direction *Food/Mood/Activity Log*s provide is only as accurate as the information they contain. Food logs are key to grasping the concepts and looking forward to the freedom that comes in **Find Your BALANCE** and beyond when *KIB* principles are used to keep hunger, and eating in response to that hunger, in their proper place.

Determining Your Child's Body Type

As previously mentioned, body typing, in some form, has been practised in Ayurvedic—long-established medicine native to India—and Traditional Chinese medicine for generations. Even in North America, the last half-century has produced increased interest and research in the fact that while every body has a goal of reaching homeostasis or balance in all its systems (i.e. metabolic, oxidative, digestive, endocrine), each of us has unique responses to those systems. Additionally, each of us has slightly different ways of maintaining that balance.

Over the past couple of decades, there have been many helpful and thorough surveys developed that cover the factors inherent in determining body type. For the *KIB* program, however, I wanted a survey specifically designed for children. Therefore, I gleaned from the wide range of body type research available, coupled that research with years of experience in working with children and adolescents, and developed a unique, customized survey. Appropriate for children and teens, the *KIB* survey comes complete with kid-friendly language and easy to understand instructions and interpretation.

In order to determine your child's body type, along with your child, complete the *KIB Body Type Survey* (p. 179). Score the questionnaire and determine if your child is a Carbohydrate Body Type, a Protein Body Type or a Mixed Body Type. While the *KIB* program is designed to be effective for everyone, your child's body type will influence the way you and your child walk out the *KIB* program. Take note of instructions throughout the book that pertain to one body type or another as that customized support more easily helps your child achieve a healthy, balanced state.

Taking Healthy Measurements

The last *KIB* concept you will need to understand before beginning **Find Your BALANCE** has to do with recording your child's weight and measurements.

Reasons for taking your child's measurements:

- ❏ It is important for you to know where your child is starting. This way, you can calculate the healthy weight range you need to aim for so you will know when **Build Your BALANCE** is over and your new lifestyle is in place.
- ❏ Taking measurements is a powerful motivational tool to keep you and your child moving forward. This is a rigorous journey and you need to be able to see progress along the way. Along with measurements, photos are also helpful. *KIB* kids get excited when they have lost inches around their waist or see changes in before and after photos, so much so that they make healthy choices even when their parents are not around!
- ❏ The process of taking measurements is one way you can begin beneficial interaction with your child over his weight. It makes excess weight something that is no longer avoided, ignored or hidden—it is something that is now manageable. This is a huge step toward freedom.

KIB's viewpoint on different types of measurements:

- ❏ Calculate but do not be overly bound by, **your child's Body Mass Index.** Google "BMI for children," calculate your child's BMI and aim for a score of roughly 25 or under. Alternatively ask your doctor to calculate your child's BMI.
- ❏ Because of the difficulty in proper evaluation of BMI calculations with children who have larger frames or higher amounts of lean tissue, also **calculate waist to height ratio (WHtR)** by dividing your child's waist size by his height. This number is more helpful than BMI in determining a healthy body size. Aim for a WHtR under .5 for your child.
- ❏ Even more effective and accurate than BMI or WHtR, you may want to **measure your child's body fat percentage**. While dual energy x-ray absorptiometry and underwater weighing are considered the gold standards of assessing body fat levels, the ratio can also be determined easily and quite precisely by using a skinfold caliper. Calipers are an effective, inexpensive and convenient tool for determining body fat percentage, and well-designed ones can provide body fat estimates that average within 1-2% accuracy of underwater measurements. Depending upon age and body type, boys should aim for a body fat ratio of about 10-23% and girls 15-31%. For body fat ratio guidelines see Tanita's site at www.tanita.com/en/healthylivingforkids/. (Tanita is a manufacturer of body fat composition monitors.) Skinfold calipers can be purchased at most fitness stores and gyms or online from www.kidsinbalance.net (Resources).

Accurately recording your child's weight and various body measurements is a necessary first step in the *KIB* program. I find that many parents do not know their child's current weight or body fat ratio, usually because they do not want to embarrass or hurt their child. The fact that accurate measurements have not been taken is important information as it tells me that a parent could possibility use some help in dialoguing about weight issues, in a beneficial way, with their child. *KIB*'s recommendations help make that healthy dialogue happen.

Here—at the point of tackling what can be the challenging task of taking measurements—is where you can step into one of your strongest parental roles: a provider of balance. Even if you do not mention it, your child knows he is overweight; he knows it because it is an everyday reality. Kids at school have no problem bringing it up, only they usually do it negatively, in a way that exposes your child to ridicule and pain. You have the opportunity to be the balancing factor in this equation; you can bring positive talk and truth to the dialogue to counteract the negativity.

Start by helping your child accept where he is right now—the measurement process can put that in motion. Before you take these measurements, think through how you can present this activity to your child. Practice a few lines to say, and play around with them until you find something that is truthful, works well and feels comfortably natural.

You may find there is still some resistance or reluctance from your child to go through this process. You may, as a result, struggle with fear and guilt about proceeding. I encourage you to gently push those fears to the side, take a deep breath and out of love for your child, move ahead. It can be very healing and freeing for your child to no longer hide the reality of his excess weight from you. Together, you can face this issue and, together, no longer fear it.

Additional, helpful measurement tips include:

- ❑ Before you take measurements, make sure you are in a pleasant frame of mind, energetic, relaxed and positive. Make sure it is a good time for your child, too. If he is upset or tired, the session may not go as well.
- ❑ Take the measurements yourself. It is important that you see the number on the scale or the measuring tape—use the soft kind, as used for sewing—or a skinfold caliper. Engage in the process; your child will benefit from seeing that you are not avoiding the issue.
- ❑ First thing in the morning is the best time to take measurements, but make sure it is a time that you can repeat in the future, as you will be re-doing this process throughout the *KIB* program. Subsequent measurements should be taken at the same time on the same day of the week (i.e. to avoid weight fluctuations due to weekend Sometimes Foods intake or days with regularly scheduled higher levels of activity).
- ❑ Prepare yourself emotionally. Seeing the numbers can be very discouraging; it is one thing to know your child carries excess weight, it is a whole other thing to find out that your 10-year-old weighs as much as an adult. If the numbers shake you up, keep emotions reasonably in check. If, however, a few tears spill out, add a smile and tell your child you are experiencing a lot of different feelings but that the things you most want to share with him are that you are excited for this journey you and he are tackling together, and you are very proud of his desire to make such healthy lifestyle changes. In fact, plan ahead to have something to say so you are not caught off guard.

Now, move forward in confidence. You are a loving parent and you are working for the health of your child now and in the future.

20 Questions Survey

The last two weeks of **Find Your BALANCE**—the mild dietary cleanse—are an integral and essential component of the *Kids in Balance* program. If properly prepared for and undertaken, along with the benefits already mentioned, days 8-21 of **Find Your BALANCE** have the potential to produce the following changes:

- ❑ Proper appetite regulation.
- ❑ Better balanced moods and emotions.
- ❑ Increased understanding/recognition of body signals (i.e. hunger, fullness).
- ❑ Improved overall sense of wellness.
- ❑ Loss of excess inches and/or fat.

Laying proper groundwork for the last two weeks of **Find Your BALANCE**, can:

- ❑ Minimize cleanse symptoms (i.e. headaches, nausea, muscle aches).
- ❑ Enable your child to more easily comply with this part of **Find Your BALANCE**.
- ❑ Prevent a sense of dietary boredom.
- ❑ Give a sense of control.
- ❑ Provide understanding of how to respond in unexpected situations.

Because **Find Your BALANCE** is such an important component of the *KIB* program, I have included a short survey to help ensure you have completed all essential preparation tasks for the phase. I want you to succeed in **Find Your BALANCE** and in the *KIB* program overall. Being well prepared for this phase is a primary key to your child's success. Therefore, please **do not start Find Your BALANCE** until you can tick off a hearty "yes" to all the following survey questions.

Twenty Questions to Ask Before Starting Find Your BALANCE

Focus	Questions
Personal - Body	❑ Have I recorded my child's baseline weight? ❑ Have I recorded my child's baseline measurements? ❑ Have I recorded my child's baseline body fat ratio (if using a skinfold caliper)? ❑ Did I take several "before" photos of my child? ❑ Has there been discussion on how to minimize sedentary habits (i.e. reducing computer time, linking amount of TV time to amount of physical movement)? ❑ Has there been discussion on how to increase functional fitness (i.e. taking the stairs instead of an elevator, walking to school, mowing the lawn)? ❑ Have I read the information on *KIB-Friendly Supplements* (p. 196) and determined which, if any, supplements are right for my child (i.e. fibre, essential fatty acids, multi-vitamin supplement, probiotic, amino acids)? If needed, are they purchased?
Personal - Mind	❑ Have we talked with the right people (i.e. teachers, doctor, coach, extended family) to ensure they understand our family's *KIB* plan and that they will support our family's efforts? ❑ Have we completed *Food/Mood/Activity Log*s to determine food triggers and the way moods interact with food choices? ❑ Have we discussed and completed the *Finding Your Motivators* worksheet? ❑ Have we discussed and completed the *Setting Your Goals* worksheet? ❑ Are the appropriate motivators planned for or obtained and ready to be distributed? ❑ Do I have an understanding of language that builds up and have ways to practise that with my child? ❑ Have I discussed and/or role-played possible scenarios with my child where it may be difficult to make good dietary choices (see *Family Meeting Time; Communication Activity*, p. 207)? ❑ Does my child understand different healthful choices that can be made in each of those possible scenarios?

Household Preparation	❑ Are the **Find Your BALANCE** menu plans chosen and completed? ❑ Have we selected and obtained a variety of healthful **Find Your BALANCE** snacks? ❑ Has shopping been completed per **Find Your BALANCE** shopping list? ❑ Have we looked at the calendar and picked an appropriate start date for **Find Your BALANCE**? ❑ Is the *KIB How Am I Doing? Chart* posted on the fridge and ready to be completed each day (p. 221)?

How did you do? If you have some boxes that are not yet ticked off then take a few more days to give yourself time to get all the essential preparation done. As I often tell *KIB* clients: you only want to **have** to do **Find Your BALANCE** once. You will likely **choose** to come back to this phase for a few days or a week or two periodically over the next few years, but if you prepare well for it the first time, it will ensure things go much more smoothly and that all the benefits **Find Your BALANCE** has the potential to produce are achieved as successfully as possible. If all 20 questions are ticked then "Congratulations!" are in order and you are ready to move on. You and your child can begin **Find Your BALANCE** now.

KIB Stories for Life

I do have an update for you . . . Hope's jeans were all getting too big so we went shopping tonight. We weren't sure what size to try so she went into the changing room with a 10 and a 12 (she was a 14 before). She came out of the dressing room with the biggest smile on her face and showed me that the 10 was too big!!! She left with a size 8 . . . and a glow of confidence and pride that I haven't seen before!!! Thank-you so much for this program. It has changed our lives and is something that we can stay with forever.

All the best.
Jane

Chapter 11

Phase 1—Find Your BALANCE

Perseverance is not a long race; it is many short races one after another.

Walter Elliott

Once you have completed preparation for **Find Your BALANCE**, the next step in helping your child move toward an appropriate body weight is a gentle cleanse. A cleanse dietary plan—one that eliminates sugars, refined grains and processed food, and instead emphasizes vegetable-source carbohydrates and healthy sources of protein and fat—goes a long way in assisting the body to break sugar addiction, begin general body house cleaning, correct blood sugar imbalances and ensure proper digestion and metabolism of food.

For most *KIB* families I suggest a three-week **Find Your BALANCE** phase—one week of gradual dietary and lifestyle modification and two weeks of dietary cleanse. (Check with your health care practitioner if you have concerns about your child doing a dietary cleanse.) *KIB's* seven solutions to a healthy weight are easy, but because they are new and far-reaching, transition can produce a bit of a learning curve. Therefore, the menu plans, recipes, and suggestions that are part of **Find Your BALANCE** are designed to provide the encouragement and practical help you and your child will need to reach your health goals.

Find Your BALANCE is both dietary and lifestyle related. Key, however, is week one's slow but sure BALANCE changes and then the creation of the menu plans needed for the last two weeks of **Find Your BALANCE**. By the time you finish reading this chapter, you will be able to easily decide which of the menu planning options described best fits your family situation, will be ready to increase both water intake and functional fitness, and will be well on your way to a successful completion of **Find Your BALANCE**.

Starting Find Your BALANCE

After a week of preparation for the *KIB* journey, it is time to begin **Find Your BALANCE**. As with your week of preparation, **Find Your BALANCE** also has its own helpful *Day-at-a-Glance Guidelines* with tips on how to cover all of *KIB's* BALANCE factors each day. The guidelines continue to help keep things simple and focused. Looking at **Find Your BALANCE** with a broader view, however, as in your preparation for this phase, there are four simple steps to **Find Your BALANCE** as well.

1) Create a menu plan for Find Your BALANCE.

Once you have finished your week of preparation, it is time for the three weeks of **Find Your BALANCE**. The first week of **Find Your BALANCE**, you will make gradual modifications in diet and exercise per the *Day-at-a-Glance Guidelines*. For the final two weeks of **Find Your BALANCE**, you will, as a family, determine to either a) get ready to eat very simply (i.e. grilled or roasted meats, legumes or nuts, and vegetables) using recipes that you and your child are already familiar with; or b) be prepared for a little more work and fill your menu plan with *KIB* Recipes following the sample *KIB Find Your BALANCE Menu Plans* (www.kidsinbalance.net/kib-resources-1.html); or c) using the concept of the protein and vegetable combinations in the sample menu plans come up with your own personalized menu plan of *KIB* Recipes; or d) do a little of all three (i.e. on busy nights do simple grilled meat and vegetable stir fries; when you have a little more time, try a few new, "That looks good!" recipes).

2) Ready. Set. Cleanse.

Proper preparation before **Find Your BALANCE** makes it much more likely that, once you begin this phase's simple, healthy dietary cleanse plan, the following benefits will occur:

- ❏ Cleanse symptoms are minimized.
- ❏ Physical or emotional addiction to certain types of food is more gradually resolved.
- ❏ Blood sugar spikes become normalized in a more gradual manner.
- ❏ Food's comfort factor is recognized and reduced in a more controlled way.
- ❏ Proper mealtime ingredients and snacks are in the house so the "failing to prepare, thus preparing to fail" factor is accounted for and eliminated.
- ❏ Recognition that healthy choices can be made and impulses can be controlled is heightened.

A simple cleanse can facilitate a growing sense of understanding—in both you and your child—that lifestyle truly can be changed. And, as positive results are attained, along with that comprehension comes pride. Done short term, a mild dietary cleanse is one of the most effective ways to safely begin transition from obesity and ill health to a more balanced state of wellness.

3) Make full use of *KIB's Food/Mood/Activity Log.*

In preparation for **Find Your BALANCE** you used the *Food/Mood/Activity Log* to record your child's dietary intake, activity and moods. Once in **Find Your BALANCE** you will continue to record those same details, but, as well, will be examining the relationship between food and your child's mood and physical responses in greater depth. Both you and your child will be introduced to four key *KIB* Food Intake Tools:

- ❏ Appropriate **Food Pairing.**
- ❏ Eating for **Comfortable Fullness.**
- ❏ A correctly balanced **Fuel Mix.**
- ❏ Good **Food Timing.**

As your understanding of these tools grows and your child more often implements them in her daily food choices, you will be easily able to use the *Food/Mood/Activity Log* to see where changes in food choice or timing, portion size or food ratios need to occur. As you and your child work to fine-tune her daily food intake, you will see increasingly positive physical and emotional responses.

4) Monitor your child's responses.

When completing your child's *Food/Mood/Activity Log* in preparation for **Find Your BALANCE**, you would have had a beginning understanding of patterns of physical and emotional responses to different foods. You may have noted fatigue or diminished mental alertness or moodiness and irritation after eating certain food types. There may have been intake of certain foods that increased energy or improved your child's mood.

In **Find Your BALANCE**, you continue to monitor your child's physical and emotional responses, particularly in four key areas:

- ❑ Bloating.
- ❑ Lack of mental clarity.
- ❑ Physical lethargy or fatigue.
- ❑ Moodiness or blues.

In **Build Your BALANCE** these four responses will be used to help you fine-tune your child's Fuel Mix. In light of the fact your child is embarking on a mild cleanse, however, during **Find Your BALANCE** the above four responses, along with skin rashes, headaches, nausea, changes in odour or consistency of bowel movements and flu-like symptoms can be indications of cleanse effects or food intolerances.

If the symptoms are effects of the cleanse, they should begin to diminish within a couple of days—note ways to minimize cleanse effects to follow (p.90). If food intolerances are contributing to symptoms, remove the food type that seems to be problematic—often dairy, eggs or peanuts—and see if there is improvement. If any of the four key responses, bloating; lack of mental clarity; physical lethargy; or moodiness continue after other cleanse symptoms have subsided, check *Fuel Mix Guidelines* (p. 187) for probable cause.

Creating a Find Your BALANCE Menu Plan

A significant part of preparation for **Find Your BALANCE** was coming up with transitional meal and snack ideas, per *Day-at-a-Glance Guidelines*, for your first week of this phase. As important as that task was, however, building a **Find Your BALANCE** menu plan for you and your child to follow during the last two weeks of this phase is even more essential. Start by ensuring you have a concrete grasp of *KIB*'s Eat for Health chapter (p. 59). Then read the additional information on Food Pairing, Comfortable Fullness and *Portion Size Guidelines* that follows in this chapter. You will need to have a good understanding of these *KIB* principles in order to create your menu plan and write out your weekly shopping list.

There are four ways to create a **Find Your BALANCE** menu plan. The easiest, **Find Your BALANCE**-Simple, is grasping the role that protein-rich foods, healthy fats and fibre play in ensuring Comfortable Fullness; taking a good look at the *Healthy Foods List (Find Your BALANCE)* worksheet (p. 217); and then using that information to slot easy, familiar meals incorporating those foods into a *Weekly Menu Plan Template* (p. 218). Follow **Find Your BALANCE** principles of having a small amount of high quality protein-rich food and fat at each meal and snack, and vegetables with most meals (i.e. recommended but optional at breakfast) and snacks per Menu Plan Guidelines below. Draw from your family's own collection of recipes and choose simple grilled or baked meats, poultry and fish or bean dishes and pair them with salads and steamed and baked vegetables that are already your child's favourites.

Secondly, you can browse through *KIB*'s Recipe section and input 14 days of new recipes into two *Weekly Menu Plan Templates* (p.218). Ensure the recipes meet the protein/vegetable requirements, enlist family help with the learning curve of multiple new recipes and enjoy the different taste sensations. Thirdly, if you like the idea of all new recipes but want help coming up with the plan, go to www.kidsinbalance.net/kib-resources-1.html and download a couple of sample weekly menu plans that make use of *KIB* Recipes.

Lastly, you can free-style it! That means creating a menu plan that includes some family favourites that work within the protein/vegetable requirements as well as including a few new recipes to try on an evening when there is more time or inclination. Whichever way you choose, have the *Healthy Foods List (Find Your BALANCE)* be your main point of reference. In order for food items to be part of your dietary plan for the last two weeks of **Find Your BALANCE**, those items have to be on the *Healthy Foods List (Find Your BALANCE)*.

Find Your BALANCE Menu Plan Guidelines

Meal	Day 1	Day 2	Day 3	Day 4	Day 5	Day 6	Day 7
Breakfast	1 protein 1 veggie	1 protein 1 veggie	1 protein 1 veggie	1 protein 1 veggie	1 protein 1 veggie	1 protein 1 veggie	1 protein 1 veggie
Snack	1 protein 1 veggie	1 protein 1 veggie	1 protein 1 veggie	1 protein 1 veggie	1 protein 1 veggie	1 protein 1 veggie	1 protein 1 veggie
Lunch	1 protein 2 veggies	1 protein 2 veggies	1 protein 2 veggies	1 protein 2 veggies	1 protein 2 veggies	1 protein 2 veggies	1 protein 2 veggies
Snack	1 protein 1 veggie	1 protein 1 veggie	1 protein 1 veggie	1 protein 1 veggie	1 protein 1 veggie	1 protein 1 veggie	1 protein 1 veggie
Dinner	1 protein 2 veggies	1 protein 2 veggies	1 protein 2 veggies	1 protein 2 veggies	1 protein 2 veggies	1 protein 2 veggies	1 protein 2 veggies

Why Cleanse?

Most of the clients I initially see in my nutritional practise—both children and adults—eat a relatively high percentage of refined grains and sugars, contributing factors to obesity and a host of other ailments. A mild cleanse or detox program eliminates refined grains and sugars, helps clients wean from sugar addictions, minimizes the negative impact of those empty calories on wellness, and moves clients toward optimal health.

Over 50 years ago, in an effort to determine when a food was food and when it became a poison, Dr William Coda Martin adopted the classical definition of a poison as, "any substance applied to the body, which causes or may cause disease." In his examination of the results of refined sugar consumption on the body, he became the first to publicly label sucrose—one form of sugar—a poison. While his remarks may have shown him as thinking outside the typical health model of that time, his evaluations were solidly based on his understanding of the medical and physical ramification of sugar ingestion.

The processing of sugar cane or sugar beets, in order to create refined sugar, strips the natural plant material of vitamins, minerals and enzymes that would naturally help our bodies process that food substance. Instead we are left with a denatured, empty or naked carbohydrate that requires vitamins and minerals from other food sources in order to digest, detoxify and eliminate the sugar.

In a very simplified explanation, refined sugar acts as a type of toxin in our bloodstream. If eaten on a regular basis or in sufficient amounts, the increased blood sugar (i.e. glucose) levels that high sugar intake produces can result in serious problems. And because natural responses to high sugar intake can create critical health challenges, the body has been designed with a built-in safeguard mechanism to defend itself against continuing high blood sugar levels. When blood sugar levels are high, the body secretes insulin, which converts excess glucose into fat and stores it in cells for later use.

Because today's intake of refined sugars makes up a higher percentage of our daily food intake than in any previous generation, it has forced our bodies to produce much greater quantities of insulin than any previous generation. As a result, we are experiencing the phenomenon of insulin resistance that in turn can lead to further health complications such as type II diabetes.

Many suffering with insulin resistance experience almost perpetual hunger and sugar cravings, particularly cravings for refined sugar. The high blood sugar levels that refined sugar intake produces set in place the body's need to reduce that blood sugar by converting it to triglycerides, a storage form of fat. Ironically and unfortunately, in an insulin resistant person, refined sugar can also become one of the few foods that gives a brief energy stimulus before that fat conversion. In this cycle, the sufferer is being chemically driven to eat more and more to achieve less and less energy production and consequently will experience weight gain that can easily lead to obesity.

Sugar Detoxification

In a sugar detox the goal is to eliminate the significant presence and effects of excess simple sugars, and thereby reset balance in blood sugar and insulin levels. Found in products such as white breads, pastas, white rice, candy, sodas, most cereals and juices, these simple sugars have had fibre and nutrients stripped away during processing. Because simple sugars metabolize quickly in the body and cause a sharp rise and equally dramatic fall in blood sugar levels, they can create a variety of imbalances (i.e. hormonal, energy, mood, pH levels).

In a sugar detox, these simple sugars are replaced with foods that require the body to work harder and longer to metabolize them and that therefore cause a more gentle elevation in blood sugar levels. These foods include fibre-rich vegetables and protein-rich foods. Modest but regular intake of healthy protein-rich foods and vegetables keeps blood sugar levels balanced, with one of many results being that the body experiences a steady energy and feeling of satiation or Comfortable Fullness all day long. As a result, the body's craving for simple sugars begins to decline, often as early as two to three days into the detox.

The process of sugar detox is a crucial way to begin a transition to a healthier lifestyle. After detox, your child's body, which up to this point has likely been working against her in matters of cravings and energy level, can now begin working with her.

KIB Food Intake Tools

In preparation for **Find Your BALANCE**, you and your child used *Food/Mood/Activity Log*s to determine if there was correlation between type or timing or amount of food and certain physical or emotional results. Now that you are in **Find Your BALANCE** you will move to a more pro-active approach and purposely implement four key *KIB* food intake tools to produce the most positive body and mind responses.

Appropriate Food Pairing—Food Pairing refers to the practise of combining a nutrient dense, long-burning food with a bulky, fibrous food to promote blood sugar stabilization, a lasting sense of fullness and an increased sense of satisfaction after eating. Foods that fall into the nutrient dense, long-burning category include animal or vegetable protein-rich foods (i.e. meats, poultry, fish, eggs, legumes, nuts, seeds, dairy) and healthy fats (i.e. nuts, seeds, nut butters, olive oil, butter, avocado). Bulky, fibrous foods include raw or cooked vegetables and, in **Build Your BALANCE** and beyond, can also include whole grains, starchy vegetables and fruit. Each time your child eats a meal or snack, she should ensure her food intake is properly paired with at least a small portion of protein and/or fat **and** vegetables.

Eating for Comfortable Fullness—Per *Portion Size Guidelines* (p. 219) your child should be eating until comfortably but not overly, full. Portions of protein-rich foods should be ½-1 times the size of a palm (½ for a snack, 1 for a meal), vegetable portions should be 1-2 times the size of an outstretched hand (1 for a snack, 2 for a meal) and fat intake should be 1-3 tablespoons/day (a tablespoon is about the size of the top of a thumb from first knuckle to tip of thumb).

Once **Find Your BALANCE** is completed and your child has moved to **Build Your BALANCE**, she will also begin to include complex, whole grains and starchy vegetable servings in about the size of one or two tightly clenched fists and fruit servings about ½ that size (depending upon body type and degree of activity). If your child is consistently hungry between meals or snacks, she is likely not eating sufficient food or eating the wrong types of foods. Conversely, if your child is not yet in her healthy weight range and hits a weight loss plateau that lasts longer than a couple of weeks, it is possible that she is eating too much food for her activity levels. Check for appropriate Food Pairing and accurate Fuel Mix to ensure satiety and balanced blood sugar levels. If your child is not satisfied nutritionally or is dealing with fluctuating blood sugar levels, the hunger signals triggered to restore blood sugar levels could be contributing to overeating.

Accurate Fuel Mix—All body types need protein-rich foods, healthy fats and complex carbohydrates in the form of vegetables. In addition, some body types have a higher need for complex grains or starchy vegetables and fruit. Be sure you know your child's body type and are helping her fuel with the correct percentage of protein-rich foods, vegetables, healthy fat and, depending upon body type and *KIB* phase, complex grains, starchy vegetables and fruit. A correctly balanced Fuel Mix best stabilizes blood sugar levels, gives sense of satisfaction and creates Comfortable Fullness. For additional information see p. 187, *Fuel Mix Guidelines*.

Good Food Timing—The concept of timely food intake comes in three parts. Because of the importance of eating before blood sugar levels get too low, the first reference is to how often your child eats each day. When blood sugar levels plunge, the body sends out urgent hunger signals. Those signals make it difficult for your child to pursue good food choices as to food type and quantity. While some people do fine eating just three times a day, many of your family members, especially children, will need to eat at least one small, properly Food Paired snack in between meals. Because eating more regularly means having a ready supply of healthy food on hand, be sure you have menu planned and grocery shopped. The biggest challenge many *KIB* families face is knowing what foods to grab quickly when time is short. Be prepared (i.e. have raw vegetables washed and ready in the fridge and snack sized bags of trail mix in the cupboard). That means there will always be a healthy snack or ingredients for a *KIB* meal available when you need them.

In addition to monitoring how often your child eats, pay attention to how much time your child gives herself after a first helping before determining whether or not she has reached Comfortable Fullness. Be sure your child waits 10-15 minutes after finishing her first plate of food. She needs to give her digestion process at least that long in order to have an accurate assessment of whether she has reached Comfortable Fullness. If she is comfortably full, she is done eating for that meal or snack. If your child still feels hungry, then she should have an additional small amount of each of the food components that make up her individual fuel mix.

Finally, be sure your child takes time at meals and snacks to thoroughly chew her food. Chewing food well aids the digestive process and slows down the pace of meals so there can be greater enjoyment of the flavours and experience of eating healthy, tasty food.

Find Your BALANCE FAQs

Q: Does my child have to follow the recommended dietary plan exactly as given?

A: Our bodies are created in a miraculous manner and they generally respond positively to any measure of improved nutrition, exercise and supplementation. It stands to reason, however, that the more completely you and your child keep to **Find Your BALANCE** recommendations, the quicker, more positive and more far-reaching the benefits. If you can adhere well to guidelines, especially the second week of **Find Your BALANCE,** so much the better. Conversely, when a plan is so strict that it seems impossible to follow, it is better to allow change to happen on a more gradual basis or to follow the plan as well as possible, but allow for a set amount of exceptions (i.e. a daily serving of fruit or starchy vegetable). While improvement will happen at a slower pace, the changes—improved levels of energy, wellness and mental clarity, improved lean tissue to fat tissue ratio—will still be very positive and are significantly better than abandoning all helpful choices.

Q: Why do cleanse effects often occur when one begins a healthy nutrition program?

A: Introducing foods or supplements of a higher and/or more healthful quality can often precipitate physical, emotional and mental detoxification symptoms. The combination of supplying proper nutrients to the body to make needed substances or to set important functions in place, along with reducing the intake of sugars, refined products and processed foods can often precipitate a cleansing effect. The enzymes, vitamins, minerals, good quality carbohydrates and protein-containing amino acids contained in a healthier nutrition plan allow the body to correct imbalances, rid itself of toxins (i.e. pesticides, drug residue, accumulated waste materials) and begin reproducing itself with improved results. Because that process necessitates the removal of toxins from tissue where it is stored and transportation through the lymph system and blood stream, various symptoms may occur. While the symptoms can be disconcerting, if allowed to proceed in a manageable fashion, they are generally signs of improving health.

Q: What kinds of cleansing effects can my child expect?

A: Increased wellness almost always includes cleansing the body. Because of individual differences, past history and degree of strictness with which a family adheres to **Find Your BALANCE** recommendations, signs of cleansing via the elimination organs—skin, kidneys, liver, colon and lungs—will vary. For some children there will be little effect, others may feel unwell for a couple of days. Potentially, however, your child could experience headaches, flu-like symptoms, slight fever (if your child's fever is moderate to high, check with your health care practitioner as there will most likely be a reason other than the cleanse), excess gas, runny nose, sore throat, hives, increased thirst, insomnia, canker sores, skin break out, bowel sluggishness or diarrhea, discouragement, mental fogginess, weakness, reluctance to exercise, irritability and, because of the way a healthier body can go back to attend to former conditions, a reoccurrence of old aches and pains. Hopefully no one gets **all** those symptoms, but be prepared for your child to experience several. Symptoms can last in a mild way up to 10 or 12 days and are usually worse on days 2-5 of a cleanse.

Q: How can I minimize cleanse effects?

A: First, do not start the last two weeks of **Find Your BALANCE** without doing proper preparation both before the phase and during the first week of **Find Your BALANCE**. Gradually reduce the amount of less than healthful foodstuffs and replace them with increased vegetables, good quality protein-rich food sources and water. The simplest, most effective and least problematic way to move to a wellness diet is to continue to eat less-than-healthful foods at the usual times in the day but to gradually reduce the volume of poorer-quality foods eaten at each meal or snack (i.e. 1 cookie instead of two, ½ can of pop instead of a full can, 1 cup of white pasta instead the 2). At the same time as you are reducing poorer food choices, begin increasing healthy foods (i.e. add a vegetable to the meal or snack, substitute quinoa for pasta). If you continue to gradually reduce unhealthy foods and increase better food choices, by the time you begin the last two weeks of **Find Your BALANCE** , your poor choices should have gradually been reduced to nil.

Next ensure your child is having regular bowel elimination and that transit time—time between food intake and food elimination—is short (i.e. under 24 hours). If your child needs work in that area, increase fibre and water intake. If further help is needed, talk to your healthcare practitioner about additional herbal/nutritional support.

Finally, ensure that the first few days of cleansing activity occur when your child has time for rest, short walks, fresh air breaks and if necessary, Epsom salt baths (i.e. a 20 minute soak in 2 cups of Epsom salts per tub full of hot water; shower off after bath). If cleanse symptoms seem extreme, slow down the process (i.e. have a few more days where the dietary plan includes minimal amounts of fruit and starchy vegetables to better give the body a chance to slowly adjust).

The gradual transition from refined sugar and grain intake toward increased intake of healthy, protein-rich foods, vegetables and water allows for more gradual waste elimination. This means any potential symptoms (i.e. headaches, stomach aches, skin eruptions, body aches) that may occur as your child cleanses are reduced in nature, intensity and duration.

Q: **How important is the amount of sleep my child gets during Find Your BALANCE?**

A: While sufficient sleep is important at any time, a foundational key to seeing positive cleanse benefits—controlled cravings, balanced moods, sustained energy and reduced fat storage—is ensuring your child has sufficient, high quality sleep each night. The constant factors in sleep quality are minimizing EMF exposure (i.e. removing electric clocks, electric blankets, cell phone chargers and computers from bedrooms) and ensuring a completely dark environment for sleeping. Additionally, there is the need to sleep appropriate amounts of time for the seasonal light exposure. This means more awake time for your child in the summer months—and saying yes to the "Please, please, please can I stay up and play a little more Kick the Can with the cousins?"—and earlier bedtimes (i.e. allowing for at least 9.5-10 hours of sleep a night) in the winter months and saying "No, it is time for bed now!"

Q: What benefits should my child begin to experience with positive nutritional change?

A: Most children and adults find their cleanse reactions quite tolerable and choose to bear with them because of the many improvements that become more evident each day they continue **Find Your BALANCE**. Generally, the initial benefits are somewhat intangible: greater strength, a sense of diminished stress, clarity of mind and an increased sense of well being. Thereafter, your child may find improvement in things such as digestive and immune system balance, inch loss, improvement in appearance of skin and a general increase in the body's ability to naturally restore itself. You and your child will have moved on to the increased wellness that distinguished physician, Dr. Philip Nolan once noted as "the next great advance in medicine. . . when people take charge of their own health."

DIGGING DEEPER
Fast vs. Slow Food

Documentaries such as *Supersize Me* are a great place to start the journey of understanding both the damaging effects of fast food as well as how "normal" the intake of that type of non-food has become.

For more on swimming upstream food wise, check out Barbara Kingsolver's book, *Animal, Vegetable, Miracle,* (www.animalvegetablemiracle.com), the story of her family's journey eating locally grown food. *Slow Food Nation* (Carlos Petrini) and *Omnivore's Dilemma* (Michael Pollan), present rationale and rallying cries for good, clean and fair food as well.

Pollan also has a children's version of his book—*Omnivore's Dilemma: The Secrets Behind What You Eat*—for kids over 12 that are interested in learning more about the foods they eat and the ways those foods are grown and prepared.

All are great resources to encourage you and your child to continue taking small steps of helpful nutritional change!

Find Your BALANCE : Action Plan Summary

Though the *Day-at-a-Glance Guidelines* are the most detailed tool by which to walk through each of *KIB's* seven BALANCE solutions to childhood obesity on a daily basis, it can be helpful to have an overview of what **Phase 1 - Find Your BALANCE** will look like.

When	What

During week 1 of Find Your BALANCE	❑ If you have not already done so, take measurements and do a weigh-in.
	❑ If you have not already done so, explain **Find Your BALANCE** to your child.
	❑ Mark all social events that may present food challenges.
	❑ Pick your **Find Your BALANCE** start date, taking note of social events, pace of life on different days and the fact there may be cleanse symptoms.
	❑ Review **Find Your BALANCE** FAQs (p. 89) on ways to minimize potential cleanse symptoms.
	❑ Choose a style of **Find Your BALANCE** eating plan from the following four suggestions:
	  1. Eat very simply per the **Find Your BALANCE**-Simple guidelines (p. 84).
	  2. Be prepared for a little more work and download and follow the online *KIB Find Your BALANCE -Sample Menu Plans* (www.kidsinbalance.net/kib-resources-1.html).
	  3. Look through the *KIB* Recipes (p. 121) and using the concept of the protein-rich foods and vegetable combinations in the sample menu plans come up with your own personalized menu plan.
	  4. Do a little of all three (i.e. on busy nights do simple grilled meat and vegetable stir fries; when you have a little more time, try some new recipes).
	❑ Whatever your chosen style of **Find Your BALANCE** eating plans, have menu plans, recipes and shopping lists ready to go.

Each meal of Find Your BALANCE	❑ Make notes on the meal (or snack) served, the family's responses and positive suggestions.

Each day of Find Your BALANCE	❑ Be sure your child drinks enough water (i.e. 4-5 glasses for every 50 pounds of body weight). ❑ Have your child eat 5-6 mini meals or meals/snacks a day; include protein-rich foods and vegetables at most meals/snacks. ❑ Have your child eat every 3-4 hours. ❑ Have your child move her body at least a little each day (i.e. walk, trampoline, biking, dancing).
After each meal in Find Your BALANCE	❑ Monitor for the following responses: 1. Bloating. 2. Lack of mental clarity. 3. Physical lethargy or fatigue. 4. Moodiness or blues. Remember that the above responses, along with skin rashes, headaches, nausea, changes in odour or consistency of bowel movements and flu-like symptoms can be indications of cleanse effects or food intolerances.
At the end of the second week of Find Your BALANCE	❑ Do you have a weekly motivator? Present it to your child with flourish. ❑ If you would like, check in with *KIB* by email. While I cannot respond to every email, I would love to hear how you are doing.
At the end of the third week of Find Your BALANCE	❑ Celebrate the end of **Find Your BALANCE** with flair—it is a significant family accomplishment!

KIB Stories for Life

Recently, Kerry (a close friend of the family) took Kyle shopping and he got 4 shirts and JEANS!!! He hasn't worn jeans since grade 1. He got a haircut. I barely recognized him when I came home from work. We did measurements that weekend. He's lost 7.5 inches [16.5 cm] off his waist since KIB. He is so motivated now. It has shifted from me to him. Your program has been so powerful for us. THANK YOU.

Anne

Chapter 12

Phase 2—Build Your BALANCE

It takes a lot of courage to release the familiar and seemingly secure, to embrace the new. But there is no real security in what is no longer meaningful. There is more security in the adventurous and exciting, for in movement there is life, and in change there is power.

Alan Cohen

Once you and your child have completed **Find Your BALANCE**, it is time to be welcomed to *KIB*'s second phase, **Build Your BALANCE**. This is the phase where additional forms of complex carbohydrates (i.e. fruit, starchy vegetables) can be carefully moved back into your child's dietary plan as you begin to better determine the fuel mix that works best for your child. **Build Your BALANCE** will last longer than **Find Your BALANCE,** but it allows your child to continue to successfully move toward a healthier, more balanced body.

Phase 1—**Find Your BALANCE**, though simple to follow, takes concentration and determination. Successful completion of that phase, however, means your child's body has become less dependent on refined sugars and grains, is more familiar with a healthy selection of protein-rich foods and vegetables, and is better balanced in terms of blood sugar levels. You are now ready to begin adding in foods that are healthier forms of grains (i.e. quinoa), and sugars (i.e. starchy vegetables, fruit).

As new as the cleanse and dietary concepts in **Find Your BALANCE** may have been for you and your child, they play a vital role in your child reaching and maintaining a healthy body size. The positive choices made over the last two weeks of **Find Your BALANCE** have potential to produce a range of healthful responses in your child's body. In turn, those healthful responses will act as important motivational tools to keep you and your child encouraged through the next phase of the *KIB* program. Here are some of the potential changes your child may have experienced thus far:

> ### How Long Does Phase 2 Last?
>
> **You cannot predict how long your child will be in Build Your BALANCE. While factors such as the amount of unnecessary weight your child is carrying and the completeness with which you follow Build Your BALANCE recommendations certainly influence duration of *KIB*'s second phase, ultimately each child's body has its own story in this regard.**

- ❑ Increased energy.
- ❑ Reduction in energy dips between meals.
- ❑ Comfortable Fullness for longer periods between meals and snacks.
- ❑ Less gassiness and gut bloating.
- ❑ A loss of 2–8 pounds or at least no new weight gain.
- ❑ Major reduction in cravings for sugary foods.
- ❑ A growing sense that he and you are in control, and that you can do this!

Starting Build Your BALANCE

One of the first things parents and children often ask before beginning this phase of the *Kids in Balance* program is, "How long does **Build Your BALANCE** last?" In short, the amount of time a child spends in **Build Your BALANCE** is very individualized. Its duration is decided both by things within your child's control (i.e. the lifestyle choices he makes during this phase) as well as by things that are beyond your child's control (i.e. the rate at which his body continues to shed excess fat). For children that have a smaller amount of excess weight to shed, **Build Your BALANCE** could last 1½-2 months. With their week's worth of preparation, 3 weeks spent in **Find Your BALANCE** and another 6-8 weeks in **Build Your BALANCE**, these children would be right on target to move into **Keep Your BALANCE**—a phase that helps maintain the health that has been achieved—in roughly 12 weeks.

For children that have a lot of weight to lose, however, **Build Your BALANCE** could last 9 months, a year, or even more. That means the same 4-week combination of preparation and **Find Your BALANCE** but an extended **Build Your BALANCE** phase. Families in this scenario would continue following **Build Your BALANCE** guidelines for a longer period of time—their 12 weeks could stretch to 12 months—but they too would eventually reach **Keep Your BALANCE** and successfully complete the program.

In **Build Your BALANCE** there is no longer the need for the structured focus of *Day-at-a-Glance Guidelines*. By now, vegetable chopping, egg scrambling, walking to the playground and getting to bed at a reasonable time will hopefully have become the norm in your home, and language like Food Pairing, Comfortable Fullness and PACEing will be familiar household terms.

As with **Find Your BALANCE**, **Build Your BALANCE** introduces a number of important simple steps. To follow, you will find those steps and explanations for critical components of **Build Your BALANCE** (i.e. appropriate amounts of activity, Intentional Eating, weight loss plateaus).

1) Continue progress with weight loss.

The primary objective in **Build Your BALANCE** is, by making healthy diet and lifestyle choices, to steadily move your child closer to an appropriate size. Reaching a balanced state is not judged solely by a number on the scale but rather is a combination of several factors which include calculating your child's WHtR (waist to height ratio; target is less than .5); BMI rating (approximate target is less than 25); taking and comparing body measurements; determining body fat ratio via a skinfold caliper or body fat weigh scale (optional but accurate and very helpful); and simply observing your child's physical state.

Though there can be a relatively quick drop in weight during **Find Your BALANCE**, weight loss slows, usually to an appropriate 1-2 pounds/week, in **Build Your BALANCE**. This is a healthful rate of weight loss that, provided there is the right ratio of energy intake (i.e. body type appropriate calorie intake) and expenditure (i.e. calories burned in a variety of ways), produces the desired loss of fat tissue rather than lean tissue. At some point, however, your child's weight loss rate will slow even further, and as long as you are consistently applying **Build Your BALANCE** dietary and lifestyle factors, it is the body's signal that it is in a balanced place and ready to move to **Phase 3 - Keep Your BALANCE**.

2) Up the activity levels.

As your child's weight continues to drop through **Build Your BALANCE**, an additional step you will need to take is to begin increasing his activity levels. Because it is much easier to get a child, or an adult for that matter, interested in becoming more physically active once he has shed some extra weight, introduce increased exercise on a gradual basis. While your child hopefully maintained his pre-*KIB* level of activity during **Find Your BALANCE**, and may even have increased his functional fitness, as weight continues to be shed (i.e. 10-15 pounds), you will now make more concerted effort to begin stepping up all three types of exercise—functional fitness, moderate intensity/longer duration and higher intensity/shorter duration—with your child.

3) Introduce Intentional Eating.

The third step in **Build Your BALANCE** is to help your child remain purposeful in his food intake choices. That entails the addition of another food intake tool for this phase—Intentional Eating. The last two weeks of **Find Your BALANCE**, you used a very specific menu plan. While you will want to continue with menu planning and use of a shopping list to ensure you have healthy meals and snacks available at all times, the **Build Your BALANCE** food plan is more flexible. With its allowance for starchy carbohydrates, as well as—after about 4 weeks—the option of a limited amount of Sometimes Foods, the increased number of variables can sometimes cause families to be less consistent in their planning. By following Intentional Eating guidelines (p. 98), you can ensure you and your child stay steady on the course toward optimal health.

Appropriate Amounts of Exercise

Because the *Kids in Balance* program is designed to manage the seven primary contributing factors to childhood obesity, **Build Your BALANCE** recommendations continue to include:

- ❑ Eating for body type.
- ❑ Having a positive attitude.
- ❑ Dealing with emotional food connections.
- ❑ Getting enough play, sleep and water.
- ❑ Sourcing quality food and avoiding non-foods.

When those factors are all being addressed, the principle of reaching a healthy weight range can pretty well be reduced to its simplest formula—weight loss occurs when we take in less energy through food volume than is expended through activity. That foundational truth, however, can lead to weight loss occurring in an unhealthy and unintelligent manner, or weight loss occurring smartly and healthily.

The *KIB* program is designed to provide the emotional, mental and physical tools to help your child take in proper and sufficient nutrients each day to provide for correct growth and development. The *KIB* factor that needs to be partnered with that food intake each day, however, is **Activity**—establishing adequate levels of physical exercise to create the energy deficit that allows for consistent, healthy weight loss. The amount of activity needed for each child will vary, but in general, if your child is utilizing *KIB* principles of Food Pairing and Food Timing; eating to Comfortable Fullness; following body type *Fuel Mix Guidelines*; and losing 1-2 pounds of body fat per week, he is doing sufficient amounts of physical activity.

If your child is following *KIB* food intake and lifestyle principles and his weight, however, has hit a plateau for more than a couple of weeks (see p. 100 for information on how to handle weight loss plateaus), it is time to increase exercise. See chapter 6 - **Activity** for additional suggestions, but in short, ensure your child's physical activity is taking place in three primary ways:

- ❑ **Functional fitness**—Look to increase physical exertion over the normal course of a day's activities. Walk your elementary-aged children to school, plan a family swim night rather than a family video night, give your child more physically active chores (i.e. mowing the lawn) and, instead of giving your teen a ride everywhere, have him walk to the pool or to friends' houses.

- ❑ **Longer duration/moderate intensity exercise**—The method of keeping fit that often comes to mind when we first think of the word exercise, aerobic activity done for a longer period of time, at moderate levels of intensity, is something your child should be doing 2-3 times/week. Longer duration/moderate intensity exercise brings with it a range of health benefits and, because it is a component of commonly found activities such as dance classes, drop-in fitness programs and community basketball and ball hockey leagues, it should be easy to find an enjoyable way for your child to engage in this important exercise form. Even simple activities like skipping rope or going on a neighbourhood bike ride will fit the bill!

- ❑ **Shorter duration/higher intensity exercise**—Done for roughly 12-20 minutes, 2-3 times a week, higher intensity exercise has many benefits. It can be easier to fit into a busy family schedule, kids usually like the interval training aspect of moving from resting to working pace throughout the activity, it causes the body to burn fat at a higher ratio for several hours after the workout, preserves lean tissue while causing extra fat to be burned and can easily be adapted to many types of activity that children love. Get out the skipping rope, dust off the trampoline or rebounder, set up a walk/run course through your neighbourhood or arrange a hilly bike ride. Whichever you choose, you will accomplish a lot of exercise benefit in a relatively short period of time. (For more information, purchase Dr. Al Sears' book *PACE: The 12-Minute Fitness Revolution* at www.kidsinbalance.net - Resources.)

Remember, your objective is not to create a skinny child; your objective is to help your child move into a healthy weight range (i.e. under .5 on the WHtR scale, under the 85th percentile on the BMI chart or into the right body fat ratio range—depending upon age and body type, between 10-23% for boys and 15-31% for girls).

Sometimes when a child meets the healthy weight range criteria he still has some excess girth around his belly. If this is your child's situation, take signals from his other physical measurements that the **Build Your BALANCE** dietary factors have done much of their work. Now it is time to focus on lifestyle factors such as continuing to monitor daily activity and ensuring sufficient quality sleep, and letting your child grow into taking increasing charge of his body. With your child's growth spurts, hormonal changes and decisions to choose to be more active, your job becomes more to support results and to encourage your child's choices each day for a healthy life.

Intentional Eating

In addition to **Find Your BALANCE**'s food intake tools of Comfortable Fullness, Food Pairing, Food Timing, and Fuel Mix, **Build Your BALANCE** makes use of a fifth tool called Intentional Eating. With **Find Your BALANCE** behind you and your child, it can be easy to drop that phase's careful planning and slip off track, but it is important to continue to be very **intentional** about what your child eats. Maintaining diligence in **Build Your BALANCE** means you can more quickly and easily move into **Keep Your BALANCE**. That, in turn, means you can be less focused on things such as vegetable intake and more focused on other parts of your lives.

Though Intentional Eating is largely a tool your child will need to embrace, the concept requires thoughtfulness on your part as well. For both of you, Intentional Eating means:

- ❑ You think big picture; eat with your end goal in mind.
- ❑ You plan ahead; preparation is insurance toward success.
- ❑ You maintain balance; create menus that look at balancing food group consumption over the course of a day and throughout a week.
- ❑ You prepare for challenges; problem solve events that may test your child's ability to make good choices.
- ❑ You remember body type; focus on foods that are the best friends of your child's body.
- ❑ You use Food Pairing and watch the order in which you eat food; it can be a good idea to start with protein, especially with Protein Body Types.
- ❑ You say "No!"; continue to avoid foods that are obvious detractors from your objectives.
- ❑ You balance energy intake with energy expenditure; eat to maintain a healthy body weight/body fat ratio.

Creating a Build Your BALANCE Menu Plan

Though there is more flexibility and food variety in **Build Your BALANCE**, the importance of continuing to menu plan cannot be overemphasized. Even in this *KIB* phase, "failing to plan" still results in "planning to fail." Take a look at the *KIB* Food Groups included in this phase (p. 99), pull out some of your family's favourite menu items from **Find Your BALANCE**, add in a couple of new choices (i.e. *Fried Rice with Vegetables*, p. 126, or *Pears in Raspberry Puree*, p. 176) and continue to thoughtfully work to help your child reach his healthy weight.

Though **Find Your BALANCE** principles of having a small amount of high quality protein-rich food at each meal and snack, and vegetables with most meals and snacks, are still essential in **Build Your BALANCE** (and indeed in **Keep Your BALANCE** and beyond), you can now add in at least one serving of high-fibre carbohydrate (i.e. yam, rice) and one serving of fruit a day if your child is a Protein Body Type, and at least two servings of high-fibre carbohydrate and 2 servings of fruit a day if your child is a Carbohydrate Body Type. If your child is a Mixed Body Type he will start with the Protein Body Type recommendations and adjust per *Fuel Mix Guidelines* (p. 187). The key to reaching and maintaining a healthy weight is to figure out how much of each of those food groups your child requires in a day and where to place them on a day's menu.

Regardless of your child's body type, start by adding foods slowly and in small amounts. As well, begin food additions from the lower end of the Glycemic Index. (Find helpful details at www.glycemicindex.com and, in particular, take note of the FAQ information on Glycemic Load.) That means first incorporating foods that take longer to break down and that are released more slowly into the blood stream. Adding foods in this manner helps to keep your child's blood sugar levels balanced and will continue to keep moods stable, energy levels steady and cravings at bay.

Start with a small serving of lower sugar fruit such as apricots, raspberries, strawberries, watermelon, cherries, cantaloupe or grapefruit, and leave higher glycemic fruits (i.e. mango, papaya and pineapple) until your child is closer to his appropriate weight range. Make use of *KIB*-friendly whole grains such as basmati rice, quinoa and sprouted grain breads. Not only are their ingredients more natural and healthy, the high fibre and low sugar content mean they too are on the lower end of the Glycemic Load Index.

Build Your BALANCE meal components for **Carbohydrate Body Types**
Each Day:
- ❑ 4-5 servings of protein-rich foods (including dairy)
- ❑ 7-8 servings of vegetables
- ❑ 2-3 servings of high-fibre starchy vegetables and grains
- ❑ 2 servings of fruit
- ❑ 1 tablespoon of healthy fats and oils
Each Week:
- ❑ 3 servings of Sometimes Foods (after 4 weeks of **Build Your BALANCE**)

Build Your BALANCE meal components for **Protein Body Types**
Each Day:
- ❑ 5-6 servings of protein-rich foods (including dairy)
- ❑ 6-8 servings of vegetables
- ❑ 1-2 servings of high-fibre starchy vegetables and grains
- ❑ 1 serving of fruit
- ❑ 2-3 tablespoons of healthy fats and oils
Each Week:
- ❑ 3 servings of Sometimes Foods (after 4 weeks of **Build Your BALANCE**)

If your child is a **Mixed Body Type** it is usually best if he starts with Protein Body Type recommendations. After a couple days of evaluation, he may need to adjust food intake slightly (i.e. decrease his protein intake, increase his starchy vegetable intake) per *Fuel Mix Guidelines*.

In the **Build Your BALANCE** Menu Plan Template that follows, the high fibre carbohydrate (hf carb) for Protein and Mixed Body Types has been slotted in for breakfast. If your child is a Protein or Mixed Body Type and prefers to have his high fibre carbohydrate with lunch or supper, you are welcome to move the serving to that meal. However, encourage your child to have both his higher starch vegetable or grain and his fruit servings before times of physical activity—at least functional fitness such as walking to school or having an outdoor recess period—rather than before sedentary activity.

The bolded high fibre carbohydrate selections in the Sample **Build Your BALANCE** Menu Plan Template are the additional carbohydrates recommended each day for Carbohydrate Body Types (Carb BT). In addition, Carbohydrate Body Types may add in one more fruit serving a day (not noted on the menu plan), provided they Food Pair with a small amount of protein.

The template also shows the addition of three Sometimes Foods per week. These can be incorporated into your child's food intake after 4 weeks of **Build Your BALANCE**, once your child's body has grown accustomed to the newly added starchy vegetables, grains and fruit. Though the Sometimes Foods are shown on the template in the evening/dessert slot, they could just as easily be used as one of the day's snack allotments.

Sample Build Your BALANCE Menu Plan Template

Meal	Day 1	Day 2	Day 3	Day 4	Day 5	Day 6	Day 7
Breakfast	1 protein 1 hf carb 1 veggie	1 protein 1 hf carb 1 veggie	1 protein 1 hf carb 1 veggie	1 protein 1 hf carb 1 veggie	1 protein 1 hf carb 1 veggie	1 protein 1 hf carb 1 veggie	1 protein 1 hf carb 1 veggie
Snack	1 protein 1 veggie	1 protein 1 veggie	1 protein 1 veggie	1 protein 1 veggie	1 protein 1 fruit	1 protein 1 veggie	1 protein 1 fruit
Lunch	1 protein **1 hf carb** **(Carb BT)** 2 veggies	1 protein **1 hf carb** **(Carb BT)** 2 veggies	1 protein **1 hf carb** **(Carb BT)** 2 veggies	1 protein **1 hf carb** **(Carb BT)** 2 veggies	1 protein **1 hf carb** **(Carb BT)** 2 veggies	1 protein **1 hf carb** **(Carb BT)** 2 veggies	1 protein **1 hf carb** **(Carb BT)** 2 veggies
Snack	1 protein 1 veggie	1 protein 1 veggie	1 protein 1 veggie	1 protein 1 veggie	1 protein 1 veggie	1 protein 1 veggie	1 protein 1 veggie
Dinner	1 protein 2 veggies	1 protein 2 veggies	1 protein 2 veggies	1 protein 2 veggies	1 protein 2 veggies	1 protein 2 veggies	1 protein 2 veggies
Dessert	1 fruit 1 protein	sometimes snack	1 fruit 1 protein	1 fruit 1protein	sometimes snack	1 fruit 1 protein	sometimes snack

How to Handle a Weight Loss Plateau

Generally speaking, your child should be losing an average of 1-2 pounds per week. Occasionally a week may go by with a little more weight loss or even a little less. If, however, your child still has not reached his healthy weight range and has plateaued at the same weight for 3-4 weeks, several factors should be examined:

❑ Ensure your child is not skipping meals.

❑ Ensure your child is not nibbling without thinking or being presented with bottomless bowls of even healthy snacks that make it difficult to monitor portion size.

❑ Ensure water is still the drink of choice and that alternate beverages, other than an optional glass of milk a day, have not slipped back into your child's diet.

❑ Ensure goals and motivators are still doing their job, or look at spending time evaluating and revising them.

❑ Ensure your child is getting enough sleep.

❑ Ensure your child is getting adequate nutritional intake and, if you have not already done so, consider having him take a good quality vitamin and mineral or whole foods supplement, essential fatty acid supplement and probiotic supplement per *KIB-Friendly Supplements* (p. 196).

Conditions such as thyroid imbalances, bacterial gut imbalances, food intolerances, certain metabolic diseases or allergies can also make weight loss difficult for some people, and should certainly be ruled out by your child's health care practitioner.

If, however, you have double-checked the above factors, your child is eating per body type, and other *KIB* principles such as stress, sleep and attitude are being attended to, the more common reasons for weight loss plateaus are need for an adjustment in energy intake or energy expenditure.

In his book, *The Fat Loss Bible*, physical conditioning specialist Anthony Colpo gives several reasons for weight loss plateaus including changes in metabolic rate and, as ironic as it may seem, the fact some weight loss has already occurred. Colpo also gives sound counsel as to how to best break through the various factors that can play a role in weight loss plateaus.

Translated into simplified *KIB* terms, when your child loses weight, his Resting Metabolic Rate (RMR), the rate at which he expends energy at rest, begins to decrease. Lean tissue burns calories at a slightly higher rate than fat tissue, therefore there will be a slightly increased gain in calorie burn as your child's lean

---

DIGGING DEEPER
Weight Loss Plateaus

Anthony Colpo's hard-hitting—especially against those promoting theories built on junk science—but well-researched book, *The Fat Loss Bible* debunks many weight loss industry myths and instead advocates real food and appropriate amounts of exercise.

The book is geared for those interested in a lean build, and his dietary principles are in line with those for a Protein or Balanced Body Type.

Should proper portion sizes, increased activity and *KIB* lifestyle principles not move your child off a weight loss plateau, download Colpo's e-book (do not be put off by the promotion style). His simple formula for determining the amount of "healthy food" grams needed per day in order to continue proper weight loss can be a helpful tool.

tissue to fat tissue ratio positively changes. Eventually, however, that small amount of change in energy expenditure will not be enough to balance out the total weight loss he is experiencing. The bottom line is that as your child loses weight—lean tissue or fat—he has less body size to be burning calories and therefore will be utilizing less calories at rest than he did before he lost weight.

Secondly, as your child loses weight, he obviously has less excess weight to carry around each day. Carrying reduced weight equates to less energy expended through regular daily activities. Again, the positive side is that your child has lost some body fat. The downside is that with the decrease in body mass, he is using less caloric expenditure on simply moving through his day.

The way to break a weight loss plateau of this nature is by once more adjusting the difference between daily caloric intake of **body type appropriate foodstuffs** and daily caloric expenditure—having your child burn more calories through all three types of *KIB* activity, than he takes in through his healthy diet. If your child is following proper portion size and Food Pairing guidelines, eating per his body type and eating until satisfied, then he simply needs to increase his daily activity levels and weight loss should again begin to occur in regular, small amounts.

Is Counting Calories Key to Weight Loss?

Yes and no. Yes—in that even if your child eats only foods that are a good fuel mix for his body type but eats beyond Comfortable Fullness, he may still gain or fail to lose excess weight. No—in that because *KIB* advocates a natural approach to wellness and makes use of dietary and lifestyle principles that have a long history of use, calorie counting is not a helpful first line of defence against excess body fat. The goal of *KIB* is to have parents teach their child lifestyle principles that lead to health for life. This includes ensuring a child has learned to appropriately listen to his body so as to know how to adjust dietary intake, activity and other *KIB* health principles to reach optimum body size and wellness.

If your child eliminates non-foods from his diet, eats a body type fuel mix of properly paired foods until comfortably full and increases his functional fitness and activity levels, his body will generally settle to an appropriate and healthy lean tissue to fat ratio.

If your child has adhered completely to these principles, his health care practitioner has ruled out any extenuating physical conditions that could make weight loss difficult, and your child has not lost body fat for 3-4 weeks, follow weight loss plateau recommendations and increase activity levels.

Only if you and your child are having consistent problems in determining the amount of exercise needed to handle appropriate

> **To Count or Not to Count**
>
> **The term calorie was not even found in the dictionary until the mid-1800s and did not come into common use as a nutritional term until the early 1900s. In days gone by, real food and physical activity were a natural part of daily living, and calorie counting was largely an unknown concept.**
>
> **While managing food intake and activity level is an important weight control tool, having children count food intake calories and determine amount of calories utilized in exercise is quite unnatural and can lead to a less than healthy attitude toward food and/or exercise. Choosing correct portion sizes and recognizing Comfortable Fullness is a better place to start.**

amounts of food intake does it make sense to perhaps more closely look at amount of food intake (i.e. amount of carbohydrate grams in proportion to protein grams) for a season until a healthy rhythm of food intake and daily activity becomes more completely established.

Build Your BALANCE Tips for Parents and Kids

This phase is called **Build Your BALANCE** for a number of reasons, many to do with the types of actions that are required by you and your child during this phase. Here, therefore, are a few additional tips that can help you and your child stay motivated and on track.

Things parents need to know about Build Your BALANCE:

It Requires You to Hold Fast—While **Find Your BALANCE** was characterized by **intensity**, **Build Your BALANCE** is characterized by **perseverance**. The challenge will be to maintain zeal for this commitment over the coming 2-12 months (or longer depending upon the amount of excess weight your child is carrying). With the year's calendar in front of you, get your child to mark the 3-month date, the 6-month date and the 9-month date; these will be important points of achievement, and will help your child understand the length of the journey.

It Requires Ongoing Cooperation—Committing to walk this wellness journey with your child requires ongoing teamwork. Communication is essential so please talk with your child regularly to make sure the food choices are working for the two of you (i.e. food budget, taste, enjoyment, preparation time). As well, continue to discuss all BALANCE aspects of this important phase.

It Requires Attention and Effort—As has already been mentioned but bears repeating, increased physical activity is a key component of this phase. While functional fitness (i.e. walking to school, active chores) will have been an integral part of **Find Your BALANCE**, as weight loss occurs it is now important to take small, gradual and sustainable steps toward helping your child embrace a more active lifestyle. Look again at chapter 6's **Activity** section for foundational information and add longer duration/moderate intensity activities to your child's schedule.

In order to increase shorter duration/higher intensity PACE exercise, have your child pick one of his favorite activities (i.e. biking, jumping on the trampoline) and begin incorporating short periods of that activity, 2-3 times/week. Start with 10 minutes of activity and gradually move up to 20 minutes. During the activity, begin with a couple minutes of slower warm-up and then alternate several cycles of work (i.e. more intense activity) and rest (i.e. a time to recover) before ending with a couple minutes of cool down. Alternating 1-minute work/1-minute rest periods is a good place to start. Later on, vary the duration of the work periods (i.e. in a 20 minute exercise period, keep rest periods consistent—say 2 minutes—but progressively move toward a shorter work period—from 2 or 3 minutes at the start to a 30 second final work period) and the intensity of each work period (i.e. start with a slower paced work period, but increase the intensity of the work periods so the final 30 second work period is done very briskly).

As your child—and other family members—get used to this helpful form of exercise, adapt the system to other activities you enjoy so its benefits of increased lung capacity, a strengthened heart and improved ability to burn fat can be achieved whether you are hiking, swimming, playing tennis or walking the dog! And remember: increase activity levels gradually, keep your child well hydrated and be sure your child's doctor has approved an active exercise program.

It Requires Effective Tools—There are a number of helpful tools you will use throughout **Build Your BALANCE**. They include:

- Keeping the motivators effective. Check the motivators that have been agreed upon and ensure they continue to work for your child. If not, work with your child to implement new ones.
- Documenting and referring to the progress that has been made. For instance, do not throw out all of the clothes your child wore at his heaviest; keep several items as a reference. It can be very encouraging for your child to try on an old pair of sweatpants and marvel at the change.
- Keeping your menu fresh. Continue to source tasty, creative recipes and find new ideas. Every few weeks, surprise your family with a new main dish recipe, or pack something different in your child's lunch.
- Counting down to the major time markers and celebrating when they arrive. Each month is a huge accomplishment and the 3-month marker is real cause for celebration. Do a fun family activity and cook a delicious healthy meal to celebrate.
- Making use of *KIB*'s written and online resources. The information is here to support you through this journey; employing all the tools available gives you a better chance of resounding success with minimal stress.

Things your child needs to know about Build Your BALANCE:

It Requires Time— Depending upon the amount of excess weight your child has to shed, he is committing up to a year or more to this phase. The degree of completeness with which he follows the *KIB* program can shorten that time, but if he is carrying quite a high degree of excess weight, prepare for about a year to really get it done.

It Requires Commitment—He will need to carefully monitor:

- Portion sizes of starchy vegetables, grains and fruits.
- The inclusion of any form of sugar in his diet.
- Exceptions (i.e. too many servings of grains or fruit in a day, Sometimes Foods).

It Requires Attention—Though **Build Your BALANCE** is simple to implement, your child will need to pay careful attention to his food intake and activity levels:

- Carefully monitoring means that your child makes decisions based on the big picture of how frequently sugar and refined grains are occurring in his diet, and how often he skips his exercise times. It is helpful to have a month-in-view calendar in a visible spot and mark down any exceptions to clearly determine how many have taken place.
- He will work hard to keep exceptions to a minimum. During the first 3-6 months of **Build Your BALANCE** it is helpful to keep your child's Sometimes Foods within the boundaries of *KIB* Recipes or in line with the many Sometimes Foods troubleshooting ideas found in chapter 13 - **Keep Your BALANCE**. Ensure, as well, that exercise omissions are few and far between.

When you finish the *KIB* program, you will likely **choose** on occasion to do a day or two of **Find Your BALANCE** or a week of **Build Your BALANCE**. You and your child, however, only want to **have** to do **Find** and **Build Your BALANCE** once. Reaching **Keep Your BALANCE** is the target.

Build Your BALANCE FAQs

Q: What if I find my child slipping, and eating more portions of starchy vegetables, grains and fruit (or even refined sugars or grains) than are recommended for Build Your BALANCE?

A: Since the goal of **Phase 2 - Build Your BALANCE** is to put an action plan in place that will allow your child's body to release as much unnecessary body fat as possible, one of those action plan objectives is to manage your child's consumption of foods that can derail your goal. If consumption of grains, fruit and Sometimes Foods goes up and weight loss stops, you know there is an imbalance. You must adjust either your child's food intake or his energy expenditure. If, however, your child has increased activity, is going through a growth spurt or is simply tall with a large frame, it could be helpful to slightly increase his quantities of high fibre carbohydrates.

If you find your child choosing more grains or fruit than vegetables over the course of a day, help him come back to the proper balance for his body. If necessary (i.e. if sugar cravings are on the rise), you could consider a mini-cleanse and do 3-4 days worth of **Find Your BALANCE** to help everyone get back on track. It is also not a bad idea to have a **Find Your BALANCE** day here or there (i.e. a day eating only a wide variety of lower starch vegetables and healthy protein-rich foods) as it can be used to help you balance out days of heavier or imbalanced food group consumption. **Find Your BALANCE** days are also a great reminder for your child that unless he is a more extreme Carbohydrate Body Type, he does not rely on starchy vegetables, grains or fruits as a major food source. These days can happen once a week and can be a very powerful wellness tool.

Q: How do I know if my child is doing enough exercise?

A: In simple terms, if your child is eating *KIB* style and losing an average of 1-2 pounds of excess weight a week (i.e. have him hop on the scale every couple of weeks and see if it is moving in the right direction, or alternatively, measure body fat ratio with a skinfold caliper and ensure the body fat ratio is slowly moving toward the healthy range) then he is likely doing enough physical activity. Realize too that excess exercise, particularly large amounts of longer-term activity such as long distance running, can place unnecessary stress on the body—find a healthy balance.

If the excess weight has stopped coming off and your child has fallen into poor dietary habits (i.e. has started eating overly large portion sizes, is not Food Pairing or is eating unhealthy foods), the first place to start is in correcting eating style. If, however, portion sizes are appropriate, nutrient dense/fibre-filled Food Pairing is happening and only foods on the *Healthy Foods List (Build Your BALANCE and Keep Your BALANCE)* (p. 222) are being eaten, then it is time to increase the physical activity.

Q: How do I know when my child has completed Build Your BALANCE?

A: Simple steps to help you determine when **Build Your BALANCE** is complete are:

❑ Waist to height ratio (WHtR) of under 0.5.
❑ Body Mass Index (BMI) below 85th percentile and around 25. Remember to use caution with BMI scoring, particularly if your child has a large frame or a high percentage of lean tissue—instead rely more heavily on the WHtR.
❑ Body fat ratio, depending upon age and body type, is between 10-23% (boys) and 15-31% (girls). See Tanita's site—www.tanita.com/en/healthylivingforkids/—for guidelines. Tanita is a body fat composition monitor manufacturer.
❑ Though your child is maintaining the appropriate eating regime and activity levels, there is no real weight loss happening.
❑ You can see with your own eyes that your child is in a healthy place.

KIB Stories for Life

I am so excited for my daughter, and my family for that matter, for being a part of your program and of your vision for helping to make children healthier who are dealing with weight issues.

Leanne

Build Your BALANCE : Action Plan Summary

When	What
Beginning of Build Your BALANCE	❑ Take measurements. ❑ Do a weigh-in. ❑ Take body fat measurements (if using a skinfold caliper). ❑ Take photos again. ❑ Mark all social events that may present food challenges.
At the end of every week	❑ Menu plan for the next week, including snacks. ❑ On alternate weeks, check the scale to monitor weight range. ❑ Do you have a weekly motivator? Present it with flourish!
Each day	❑ Make notes on everything you serve, how it went over, what you might change. This will help you develop your own collection of workable ideas. ❑ Expand your cooking repertoire—re-work some of your favourites to fit *KIB* criteria, search online or buy a new cookbook for inspiration.
After 2 weeks in Build Your BALANCE	❑ It has been six weeks since your child started the *KIB* program—find a way to mark this achievement!
After 4 weeks in Build Your BALANCE	❑ On alternate weeks, check the scale to monitor weight range. ❑ Review your child's progress; go over **Build Your BALANCE** FAQs to be sure you are covering all the bases. ❑ Add in up to 3 servings of Sometimes Foods per week.
Upon a weight loss of about 10 pounds	❑ Look at *KIB*'s **A**ctivity material and begin gradual implementation of a more active level of all three recommended types of physical exercise (i.e. functional fitness, longer duration/moderate intensity, shorter duration/higher intensity intervals of work/rest).

Chapter 13

Phase 3—Keep Your BALANCE

A truly good book teaches me better than to read it. I must soon lay it down, and commence living on its hint. What I began by reading, I must finish by acting.

Henry David Thoreau

By the time you reach **Keep Your BALANCE**, you have helped transition your child to an appropriate body weight and are moving into a lifestyle that supports maintenance of that healthy weight. The objective in this third and final phase of the *KIB* program is for you and your child to keep up and enjoy the results you have successfully achieved. **Keep Your BALANCE** is with your family for life.

At this point in the *KIB* journey, your child is very likely enjoying consistent levels of energy, increased ability to focus, and healthy mood and blood sugar level balance. You can be proud of the fact you have helped lower your child's risk of heart disease, Type II diabetes and other health concerns associated with prolonged excess weight or obesity.

Even though your child is within healthy weight range parameters, you may feel she still carries a few unnecessary pounds. (i.e. a small roll around her waist or upper back area). Just remember, your job was only ever to get your child healthy and safe from the risks associated with excess body fat. Leave the body sculpting to time and future careful management by your child's adult self. This is a life-long journey and your child's body will continue to be positively affected, on a daily basis, by the changes you have made.

Starting Keep Your BALANCE

You and your child may find it somewhat unsettling to enter **Keep Your BALANCE**; it can be hard to relax and trust that the two of you can maintain your positive results and not slip back into old habits. The truth is, however, it is very unlikely that you and your child will ever forget where you have come from, why you wanted and needed these changes so badly and how diligently you have worked. You may have days where you will make less than healthy exercise choices or have a season of being a little off track with what you know is your child's best fuel mix, but because of your new understanding and the lifestyle you have walked out for several months, it is likely that you are here to stay.

As with the other *KIB* phases, **Keep Your BALANCE** also introduces additional important (and in this phase, quite fun!) terms: Sometimes Foods and Celebrating Well.

1) Sometimes Foods

Now that you and your child are living a newly balanced lifestyle, you will be keenly aware of the endless opportunities to partake in Sometimes Foods, foods that may be tasty and fun but are less than optimal dietary choices (i.e. because of poor quality ingredients, wrong fuel mix for your child's body type or higher degree of sugar content).

Though Sometimes Foods have been mentioned briefly in previous chapters, it is in **Keep Your BALANCE** that they take a more prominent role in a household menu plan and, therefore, where their function and impact on the body needs to be more fully explored. In **Keep Your BALANCE** you and your child will grow in understanding of what constitutes Sometimes Foods, when the best time is to partake of them and how to source the best types of Sometimes Foods.

2) Celebrating Well

In general, household menu planning, shopping and food preparation should be centered on eating body-type healthy foods in a variety and amount that maintain an appropriate weight and overall wellness. In most homes, however, the basics of family life are interwoven with celebrations—opportunities for tradition and nostalgia to create a tug at the emotional heart, that in turn prompts choices not always best for our physical heart (and other body parts).

Christmas dinner, for instance, may find a family serving marshmallow-covered sweet potatoes, a high sugar content jellied salad and white flour rolls along with the roast turkey, simply because the recipes for those side dishes have been handed down and served at holiday meals for generations. Other celebratory events—family birthday parties and movie nights for instance—may, over time, have come to be defined by bowls of candy and chips washed down by sugary drinks.

Regardless of the special occasion, what sufficient time in **Keep Your BALANCE** reveals is that our foods have strong heart connections. That means we may opt to cling to foods that are a poor wellness choice, even if our taste buds do not appreciate them any more, simply for fear that changing the food may negatively impact the emotional experience of an event. Celebrating Well helps you and your child keep the positive emotions and celebratory nature of a festive occasion, without setting off a wide range of negative responses in your child's body, mood and emotions.

Sometimes Foods

Before taking a good look at how to have healthy celebrations, it is important to have increased clarity on *KIB*'s definition of Sometimes Foods. While these foods have their place in the weekly food plan of a healthy child or teen, try to follow the 80/20 Rule—a minimum of 80% of your child's food intake should be nourishing foods her body is designed to be fueled on and no more than 20% of her intake should be Sometimes Foods. At least initially in **Keep Your BALANCE** you may want to hold Sometimes Foods to an even smaller proportion of your child's diet. She may still be working toward optimal health in other areas (i.e. skin condition, sleep patterns) or though in an appropriate weight range, may still have a small tummy roll she wants to reduce. In that case it makes more sense to keep Sometimes Foods to their **Build Your BALANCE** level—three times/week. Either way, 80/20 Rule or **Build Your BALANCE** level, in a culture that has clearly lost the meaning of "sometimes," one of the primary tasks for you and your child in **Keep Your BALANCE** is going to be handling the Sometimes Foods challenge.

KIB knows that foods often come wrapped in more than the brown paper bag or cardboard box they arrived in from the store. Food's emotional packaging can, at times, present a challenge for you and your child. Here, therefore, are some guidelines for dealing with Sometimes Foods—foods that we know are not all that good for us but that we choose, under certain circumstances, to eat anyway.

- **Look up the definition of "sometimes."** The very name for these types of foods gives you good guidelines as to how often to indulge: from time to time, occasionally, now and then, on occasion, at times. Recognizing that society has made Sometimes Foods an inappropriate multi-times-a-day occurrence is the first step to helping keep foods of this type in their proper place. When something becomes commonplace, it means the bar must be continually raised, both in quantity and level of excess, for special events. Work to keep Sometimes Foods a true exception.

- **Evaluate nutritional information.** Because an increasing number of studies show that consumption of goods high in unnatural fats—particularly trans fats—and refined sugars—particularly high fructose corn syrup and other forms of fructose—can be hazardous to health, foods containing these ingredients should be on your family's "never" or "almost never" food list.

- **Remember that Sometimes Foods are generally not good for you and are not, in most cases, even neutral.** Depending upon the type of Sometimes Foods, they can rob the body of nutrients in order to complete their digestion and metabolism (i.e. high amounts of refined sugars or unhealthy fats), contribute to constipation (i.e. refined grains and sugars, poor quality protein choices) and increase the body's toxic load (i.e. refined sugars and grains, chemicals, additives). That, in turn, means more work for your body's primary elimination organs—the liver, colon, kidneys, lungs and skin.

- **Decide when to eat Sometimes Foods.** Look at whether your family is maintaining optimal weight and health. If so, Sometimes Foods are more likely an option. Realize though that even at optimal health, some products (i.e. pop, poor quality candy, high sugar/trans fat, chemical or additive-filled foods) should probably be on a "never" or "almost never" list.

- **In general, keep Sometimes Foods off your list of motivators.** It does not make sense to reward your child with things that could potentially be harmful to her. Instead affirm positive behaviour, reward goal attainment or celebrate important events with one-on-one time, special activities or non-food gifts such as a book or game. On the odd occasion when Sometimes Foods makes it on to the list of motivators, be sure it is small amounts of high quality Sometimes Foods.

- **If you are not feeling well, avoid Sometimes Foods.** Research shows that certain foods enhance the body's ability to fight illness while others can erode the body's defence system (i.e. sugar is immuno-suppressive). When sickness or additional stress is imminent or already present, give your child's body a chance to deal with the stressors rather than offering foods that may contribute to the problem.

- **Do not use Sometimes Foods to give quick energy between errands or before physical activity.** Because refined grains and sugars are rapidly broken down by the body and released into the blood stream where they quickly elevate blood sugar levels, they can give a sense of increased energy. Their impact is short-lived, however, because the pancreas secretes insulin to reduce those high blood sugar levels. As insulin does its job, the resultant decrease in blood sugar levels can produce fatigue, irritability and mental fogginess, and trigger the body's hunger/eat mechanism so blood sugar levels can again be increased. Instead, use body-type ratios of modest amounts of healthy protein-rich foods and high fibre carbohydrates to provide the energy needed for a day at school or a sports practise.

- **Try to have Sometimes Foods that are somewhat healthy** (i.e. natural ice cream or snack foods without MSG and additives) and/or munch them with a handful of baby carrots or cucumber slices so you are getting some good nutrition with the not so great Sometimes Foods. And as for those movie night snacks or Christmas candied yams, why not see if you can find a suitable substitute (i.e. organic, fair trade dark chocolate and sparkling water with a dash of unsweetened cranberry juice), or revamp grandmother's traditional recipe (i.e. eliminate sugar, increase vegetable content, substitute quinoa for white pasta) by checking out recipes at www.worldshealthiestfoods.com; try their *Yams with Ginger and Cinnamon* or *Healthy Mashed Sweet Potatoes*. That way you can lose the less-than-beneficial health impact and keep the nostalgia.

- **Even with Sometimes Foods, practice Food Pairing.** Avoid eating grains and sugars alone. The quick blood sugar rise produced by refined grains and sugars can be somewhat moderated if foodstuffs like cookies, bagels and chips are paired with protein-rich foods. Add chopped almonds and old-fashioned oats to your homemade chocolate chip cookies, top the bagel with natural peanut butter or cream cheese and tomato slices, and have a chunk of Irish cheddar with your corn chips and salsa.

- **Check the calendar.** Look and see what is happening for that day, week and month. When your child sees there is a school party planned for Thursday it will make a simple snack of red pepper strips and a turkey pepperoni stick on Wednesday afternoon seem logical and acceptable. Even youngsters can grasp the concept that too much of a not very good thing is not very good.

- **Look to the other parts of *KIB*'s BALANCE formula** to bring stability to your intake of Sometimes Foods. For example, increase exercise and water when you know you are going to indulge, and ensure sufficient sleep, particularly in winter months, to counterbalance carbohydrate cravings.

Finally, just as in any other area of family responsibility, keep a constant eye on the big picture. Eating for health is ultimately your goal.

Celebrating Well

While you may certainly have done some celebrating during **Build Your BALANCE**, it is once your child has entered **Keep Your BALANCE** that celebration—with its usual accompaniment of Sometimes Foods—may begin to happen on a more regular basis for your child. Learning to celebrate well is a key component to maintaining ongoing optimal health.

Now that your definition of Sometimes Foods is clearer, the next step is looking at holidays and celebrations, an important part of every healthy household. In most families—particularly a family that has made significant progress toward balanced health—birthday parties, vacations and the month-long season of festivities that includes Christmas, Hanukkah or Kwanzaa (and their accompanying high-sugar, low fibre foods) can be a challenge. When following the *KIB* approach, I encourage you to work to keep the Sometimes Foods exceptions to a minimum, particularly if you hit celebration seasons during **Find Your BALANCE** or early **Build Your BALANCE** phases. Here are a few ideas to help get you through any type of celebration in a positive and healthy way:

- Discuss together as a family what you want to achieve throughout a vacation or the holidays. Identify the big challenges (i.e. dinner at Grandma's house, visiting an all-inclusive resort, a neighbourhood party) and strategize how you will handle them. You can even talk through or role-play scenarios to help your child have ready-made responses for tough moments.
- Pack portable snacks, or eat healthy foods just before attending an event that may be challenging. Keep a cooler in the trunk and load it up with great options.
- Do not skip meals—you will be hungry and leave yourself vulnerable.
- Continue drinking lots of water.
- Find a handful of tasty new green light or yellow light recipes (see *Red Light, Green Light; Label Reading Activity*, p. 205 for definition of green, yellow and red light foods) to delight your family so they are better able to say no to the red light options.
- Encourage your child to have a small portion of Sometimes Foods and enjoy seconds of the green light foods.
- Balance times of excess with increased exercise and/or with **Find Your BALANCE** days on either side of a special occasion.
- Talk, in advance, to close friends and family members who will be in attendance at get-togethers and explain to them what you are doing and why. Ask them to help out by not pushing food on your child and let them know that a hug and caring interactions are the best kind of love to express to your family. Thank them heartily for their cooperation.

In a nutshell, what you and your child are attempting to do is to redefine celebration in ways beyond simply food and inactivity. Below are a variety of suggestions to help you on the journey. Use the list as a springboard to create your own ideas of what your family could do to replace eating excessive amounts of Sometimes Foods or doing sedentary activities such as watching a movie.

- Do a family craft—even if you are not crafty. It could be extremely fun and, at the least, create unforgettable memories.
- Volunteer at a food bank or some other organization focused on giving.
- Go to the mountains or a local park and, depending upon the season, enjoy an afternoon of hiking, tubing or cross-country skiing.
- Go skating—roller or ice.
- Play active inside games such as Cadoo or charades.
- Go to local events around town—there are lots of free activities going on most holiday seasons and throughout the summer months.
- See some live theatre or a concert; though somewhat sedentary in nature you can plan to park farther from the venue and fit in a short walk before and after the event.

- If you live in a snow belt, when those flakes fall, go out and play! And don't be afraid to get your child shoveling.
- If rain is more your local climate pattern, don't let it keep you inside. Throw on boots and a rain jacket and go exploring despite the weather.

One of *KIB*'s four cornerstone beliefs is that today's commonly accepted lifestyle and cultural practices do not necessarily support reaching or maintaining a healthy weight. That belief is rarely more evident than in times of celebration. Have the courage to **not** live up to everyone else's expectations. Work with your family to set a new standard for entertaining both in volume of food intake as well as degree of inactivity.

- When entertaining, there is often underlying pressure to have food available at all times. Do not give in to the bottomless bowl practice. Serve pre-portioned snacks on individual plates, or simply put out smaller amounts of food at different times during the event.
- Suggest an evening walk with your guests to enjoy spring flowers, fall leaves or the lights and decorations during holiday seasons. Who knows? Maybe some bird watching, flower identification or spontaneous caroling will break out!

And finally, search out and serve delicious but amazingly healthy celebration recipes. Explore natural food websites (i.e. www.worldshealthiestfoods.com), healthier choice magazines (i.e. www.eatingwell.com) or check out the cuisines of different ethnic groups. Though celebrations happen pretty much world-wide, in cultures that have yet to become as caught up in excess consumption or have less access to as wide a range of processed food, people often have a better understanding of real food celebration. Their recipes and traditions usually reflect that fact.

Creating a Keep Your BALANCE Menu Plan

There are only a few dietary changes in **Keep Your BALANCE**, but they are encouraging ones. Many children can handle an extra serving of fruit a day, as well as several extra servings of high fibre carbohydrates. That means more snack variety and more options for meal planning.

Keep Your BALANCE meal components for **Carbohydrate Body Types**
Each Day:
- 4-5 servings of protein-rich foods (including dairy)
- 7-8 servings of vegetables
- 6-8 servings of high fibre starchy vegetables and grains
- 2-3 servings of fruit
- 1 tablespoon of healthy fats and oils
Each Week:
- 3-5 servings of Sometimes Foods

Keep Your BALANCE meal components for **Protein Body Types**

Each Day:

❑ 5-6 servings of protein-rich foods (including dairy)

❑ 6-8 servings of vegetables

❑ 2-4 servings of high-fibre starchy vegetables and grains

❑ 1-2 serving of fruit

❑ 2-3 tablespoons of healthy fats and oils

Each Week:

❑ 3-5 servings of Sometimes Foods

Children with **Mixed Body Types** should check their *KIB Body Type Survey* results for the body type in which they scored the second highest number of points. They can then start with the recommended number of servings of each food group for that Body Type. After a couple days of evaluation, they may need to adjust food intake slightly per *Fuel Mix Guidelines* (p. 187).

In **Build Your BALANCE**, one of the keys to your child **reaching** a healthy weight was to figure out how much of each of *KIB*'s Phase 2 food groups your child required (i.e. food quantity per *Portion Size Guidelines* and eating for Comfortable Fullness) and where to place them on the day's menu (i.e. Food Pairing, eating protein as the first part of a meal, including grain and fruit servings before exercise). The key to **maintaining** a healthy weight for your child in **Keep Your BALANCE** is similar—figure out how much of the new possible amounts of each of those food groups your child requires in a day and decide where to place them on a day's menu.

If your child is a Protein Body Type and her weight increases when you add in additional starchy vegetables, grains and fruit, either work with your child to increase activity levels or reduce serving sizes of starchy vegetables, grains and fruit (particularly gluten-containing grains: barley, rye, oats and wheat). If your child is a Carbohydrate Body Type and her weight increases when you add in more starchy vegetables, grains and fruit, ensure the grains are sprouted or move to non-gluten grains such as quinoa and rice. Ensure the carbohydrates are accompanied with sufficient vegetables and lighter sources of protein (i.e. legumes, less-fatty fish, the white meat of poultry) and that you have not too quickly increased the serving sizes of the starchy vegetables, grains and fruit. If your child is a Mixed Body Type, determine which of the Protein Body Type or Carbohydrate Body Type factors mentioned above seem most appropriate for your child and adjust accordingly.

Additionally, in **Keep Your BALANCE** continue to fine-tune type and amount of physical activity to ensure your child is able to maintain a healthy weight through growth spurts; puberty; the fact she has a lower overall Resting Metabolic Rate; and other physical or emotional transitions on the way to adulthood.

Keep Your BALANCE Tips for Parents and Kids

The biggest difference between **Build Your BALANCE** and **Keep Your BALANCE** is that the emphasis on the *KIB* program itself—this intensive time of transition—is over. Though you will continue feeding your child and your family in the healthy manner you have adopted, other family priorities can move into primary focus. Here are a few tips that can help you and your child easily adapt to that shift in direction.

Things parents and kids need to know about Keep Your BALANCE:

It Requires You to Loosen Up—While **Find Your BALANCE** was characterized by *intensity* and **Build Your BALANCE** was characterized by *perseverance*, **Keep Your BALANCE** is characterized by *freedom*. Your child is now free of excess body fat, free from increased associated health risks, free from the emotional challenges of carrying excess weight, free to live this new lifestyle with ease and free to focus on other important aspects of life.

It Requires Use of Effective Tools—Though there is a high degree of liberty in **Keep Your BALANCE** it does not mean you and your child abandon all self-control. Tools you will continue to use include:

- ❑ **Calendars:** It is helpful to mark days of excess on the calendar and plan accordingly.
- ❑ **Dialogue:** Talk often with your child to make sure her food choices are working.
- ❑ **Balance:** Balance times of excess with **Find Your BALANCE** meals and additional physical activity.
- ❑ **Experimentation:** Keep your menu fresh by continuing to source new recipes and ideas.
- ❑ **Celebration:** Do something really special to mark your success with the *KIB* approach and continue healthy celebrations together as a family.
- ❑ **Reflection:** Every now and then, pull out old photos and reflect on the journey your child has traveled. Affirm her attractiveness and inner qualities at both the start of that journey and now, and enjoy the feeling of having conquered this major life challenge.
- ❑ **Connection:** Keep in contact with *Kids in Balance*. While I cannot reply to every piece of correspondence, I would like to hear how you are doing; please feel free to send an email.

It Requires Use of Intentional Eating—In **Keep Your BALANCE**, you and your child will still practice Intentional Eating (p. 98) but by now it is much more fluid and requires less effort or focus. It is indeed a new habit. As well, continue to move forward carefully with adding in additional servings of high fiber starchy vegetables, grains and fruit. Observe how your child responds both emotionally and physically to each additional food option. Continue to check *Fuel Mix Guidelines* and remember you are looking for balance.

It Requires Evaluation—As mentioned often throughout *KIB* material, numbers are not the goal, and numbers need proper interpretation. However, for the first couple of months of **Keep Your BALANCE**, record your child's measurements and weight once a month (at the same time each month). This helps reassure both you and your child that she is maintaining the success she gained in **Build Your BALANCE**. After that, relax and let go; you can verbally check in with your child every now and then as to how her clothes are fitting, but both of you know what you need to do to stay healthy and can work to monitor that extra weight does not begin to creep back on again.

If there comes a point when your child seems to be putting on excess weight or where you are concerned that too much unhealthy food is coming back into your family's lifestyle, print off a copy of the *Food/Mood/Activity Log* and either you or your child can fill it out for a week. Observe when your child is making poorer food or activity choices and strategize to help your child find ways to better deal with those situations. For instance, if the hardest time for your child is after school at a friend's house, perhaps you can send along extra healthy snacks for her on that day.

It Requires Being Mindful of Sometimes Foods—Rather than allow intake of less healthy foods to slowly creep to a place of everyday occurrence, use the calendar, see what is on the week's schedule and help your child decide when she will have the small plate of nachos or a couple of homemade oatmeal-walnut-chocolate chip cookies. Recognize that intake of Sometimes Foods 3-5 times a week can be a part of a healthy lifestyle and making good decisions about when to have those Sometimes Foods is an important facet of **Keep Your BALANCE.**

It Requires Trust—Sometimes believing that a goal has actually been reached can be difficult. You may find yourself being overly concerned about going backwards and losing the ground that has been gained. Look at reality and accept the truth that you and your child have accomplished what you set out to do.

While you will need to be careful to shop for and prepare the foods you know will support your child's positive results and you must continue to keep regular physical activity part of your family's lifestyle, it is important to keep balance between the desire to maintain this hard-earned success and the enjoyment of your new life experience. Your child will want to take pleasure in the sensation of being an average-weight child for what might be the first time in her life. Be sure to allow room for that enjoyment to happen.

It bears repeating—if your child is in an appropriate weight range for her height and age, and her waist to height (WHtR) ratio is under .5, do not worry about a couple of pounds or a small roll around her tummy. Your job as a parent was to get your child out of risk and into a healthy range of balance. It was not to create a sculpted physique and certainly not to produce a toothpick girl. Generally, this small roll or amount of weight will be taken care of over the long term as your child maintains her healthy lifestyle. Your child is still growing and maturing; height and a sense of ownership over her physical state will increase over the next few years and contribute to ongoing balance.

Have faith. Provided you and your child maintain a **Keep Your BALANCE** lifestyle, childhood obesity is behind you.

Keep Your BALANCE FAQs

Q: Are you saying I will need to pay particular attention to what my child eats for as long as I am responsible for her care?

A: Yes. As you have learned with the *KIB* approach, what your child eats impacts her body in all manner of health and wellness ways. The Eat for Health principles of body-type appropriate Fuel Mix, Food Pairing, Comfortable Fullness and Celebrating Well are principles that, if adopted as lifestyle rather than quick fix, have the potential to provide your child with optimal mental, emotional and physical health for the rest of her life. As you have implemented and become accustomed to following *KIB*'s Healthy Living Pyramid components, your learning curve has flattened, the everyday requirements of planning, shopping and meal preparation have become easier and the wellness results have begun to appear. Continuing in a **Keep Your BALANCE** manner of intentional planning and eating is a life-long legacy well worth passing on to your child.

Q: Celebrating Well seems like a lot of work. It is o.k. simply to revert to old patterns during holidays and vacations?

A: Do not give up vacations, birthdays or holidays as lost time. You will be giving up too much. Though society often throws health and wellness caution to the wind—even more than usual—during times of festivity, teaching and modeling the concept of Celebrating Well is an amazing gift to pass on to your child. In fact, you will find your family feels better and is able to enjoy much more of life when you maintain your current lifestyle and add in only a few exceptions.

Q: **What do I do if my child does not want to celebrate well?**

A: Go through the following suggestions with your child:

- Clarify the reasons your child is feeling this way and ask her to be specific. For instance, your child may say that she will not be able to eat anything tasty over the holidays or she will feel left out of festivities.
- In a positive manner, remind your child of how great she felt when your family worked hard and she lost excess weight during **Find Your BALANCE** and **Build Your BALANCE** phases.
- Explain to your child that you believe she can enjoy flavours of the special occasion without having to have all the damaging excess or unhealthy ingredients. In fact, your goal is to have her choose and enjoy her very favourite foods. The difference, however, is that now during celebrations you will be smarter about timing, quality and quantity of food items. Explain how you will game plan with her (i.e. Food Pairing, cleanse days, planning active play) and ask her how the two of you can make this work.
- Do not give up too soon; keep questioning any assumptions and offering scenarios of how it could work until you both come to an agreement of strategy.
- Remember, children generally believe what their parents believe. Hold fast to the fact that she truly feels better in this new lifestyle and that she is on the path to getting the weight issue firmly behind her. Each celebration will be a whole new discussion, but focus on getting through the one right in front of you in a positive and healthy manner.

Keep Your BALANCE : Action Plan Summary

When	What
Beginning of Keep Your BALANCE	❑ This is a wonderful time to take some "after" photos. ❑ Check weight, waist to height (WHtR) measurements, and body fat ratio (if using a skinfold caliper or body fat weight scale). ❑ Explain **Keep Your BALANCE** to your child. ❑ Continue to mark upcoming social events; plan how to handle events. ❑ **Celebrate** as a family—you did it!
At the end of every week	❑ Menu plan for the next week, including snacks.
Each day	❑ Live the lifestyle you know best supports your child in maintaining a healthy, balanced body. ❑ For the first 3 months or so, monitor your child's response to the extra starchy vegetables, grains and fruits, and modify accordingly.
Beginning of 2nd month	❑ Check weight, waist to height (WHtR) measurements, and body fat ratio (if using a skinfold caliper or body fat weight scale). Check in verbally with your child. You want to make sure she is maintaining. Remember to account for any growth that will naturally take place in the days and years ahead.
Beginning of 3rd month	❑ Check weight, waist to height (WHtR) measurements, and body fat ratio (if using a skinfold caliper or body fat weight scale). Check in verbally with your child. If a reasonably steady state is being maintained, put away those tools of measurement and move forward confidently. If not, review your menus and your child's activity levels and adjust as necessary.
Observe	❑ Are you noticing any other changes in your child? Is she venturing into new opportunities, getting more involved or doing better in school? These changes can all be results of *KIB*'s lifestyle transitions!
Ongoing	❑ As it is easy to get into a meal planning rut, continue to occasionally expand your cooking repertoire. Take a cooking class with your child or subscribe to a healthy food magazine.

KIB Stories for Life
(Exactly as I received it and one of my all time favourites!)

Hey this is Josh,
I am very excited to say I have lost 7 ¾" [17cm] & 10 lbs [4.5kg]! I am looking forward to losing alot more, I am exercising alot!

I ride my bike 45min.every morning & alot in the afternoon (rain or shine)

I am eating more veggies than I used to . Cukes are my favorite!

Thanks for all your help and wisdom, I am just beginning Build Your BALANCE.
My Mom & Dad are helping me.some times they mess up
(ok I mess up too)

Happy Easter!
Josh (12 years old)

Conclusion

Not long ago, I had an epiphany that underscored my passion for bringing *Kids in Balance* principles to as many families as possible. Early one morning, at my nutritional consulting practise, I received a phone call from the mother of a 13-year-old with an eating disorder. The young girl had already had a two-week period of hospitalization because of the severity of her anorexia and bulimia, and had been struggling desperately with the disorder for over a year. As the mom began to recount her daughter's history, several statements stood out: she had always been a heavier child; she is a different shape than her two older sisters who never had weight challenges; even as a toddler she was always hungry; and increasing grains to give her more energy hadn't helped. As I began to explain some of the whole foods and body typing principles that are key to the *KIB* program, it was as though the mom had light bulbs going on in her head. "That makes sense." "That would explain why what we were doing wasn't helping." "Now I understand." And then finally, "Why didn't someone tell me this years ago?"

Later that day, I met with a mom and her 10-year-old daughter who had been following *KIB*'s program for four months. I was greeted with huge smiles and a plate of vegetables and healthy dip. Before the family began the *KIB* program, they had been confused as to the best way to help their young daughter shed her excess body fat but now were well versed in the BALANCE way of doing life. Their refrigerator and pantry were full of whole foods, a variety of healthy protein-rich fare was a natural part of their Protein Body Type daughter's daily diet, and exercise had become a regular part of her life. Not only was she still doing the synchronized swimming she had done pre-*KIB* but mother-daughter walks were now happening as well, and for rainy days there was a stationary bike and treadmill in the TV room for a shorter duration/higher intensity workout.

The daughter knew the best times to fit her starchy vegetable, grain and fruit servings in during the day and had learned to moderate portion size too. She had shed 19 pounds, most of it excess body fat and much of that from around her midriff. Even more importantly, this young girl had shed the right type of weight, had done it in a healthy manner and had learned lifestyle tools to last her a lifetime. No longer having to face the potentially problematic health future of an obese child, she had also been spared the heartbreak, and physical and emotional complications of disordered eating. The *Kids in Balance* program is known for the benefits it provides. That day I also soberly realized what the *KIB* program has the potential to prevent.

By the time you have reached this section of the book, you are likely a parent who has successfully helped your child complete the *KIB* program. My hope is that as you carry on your wellness journey, you will continue to delight in the amazing uniqueness of your child's body type; that you will help your child grow in his ability to choose good attitudes; that you will foster loud and frequent laughter in your home; that you will encourage regular family physical activity; that sufficient sleep and water intake will be what you model as integral components of your new lifestyle; and that you will continue to make nourishing your family an important part of your daily routine. And by nourishing, I mean you will stretch yourself to cook more from scratch, will serve fresh, wholesome foods and will make family meal times happy, rejuvenating experiences that support the health of each individual family member. If you commit to those goals, then well done—you have solved the childhood obesity puzzle and health truly is in your home!

KIB Recipes

With a firm grasp of *KIB*'s Food Fundamentals—1) eating real food, 2) eating that food as close as possible to its original form and 3) not becoming slave to any dietary plan—it becomes an easy task to organize your family's nutritional intake. Those whose bodies do better on a higher percentage of carbohydrate-rich foods will have a weekly menu plan of meals that includes daily starchy vegetable, grain and fruit intake. Those with a Protein Body Type will adjust their meal plans to include a higher percentage of protein-rich foods with mainly vegetables as their carbohydrate intake. Mixed Body Types will plan their meals to fall somewhere in the middle of a carbohydrate and protein approach. For households that include a variety of profile types, meals will contain a variety of foodstuffs that individuals can then tailor to what best suits them individually.

Think variety when planning meals. This ensures the inclusion of a wide assortment of nutrients, minimizes allergy potential and helps avoid boredom. On the other hand, you do not need to have 365 days' worth of meal plans. Most families do fine on a two or three week rotation of meals with some allowance for seasonal adjustments (i.e. more soups and stews in the winter, more salads and lighter meals in the summer). A rotation between 3 or 4 breakfast meals, 3 or 4 lunch meals, and suppers that include perhaps 2-3 poultry meals, 2-3 red meat meals, 1 fish meal and 1-2 legume meals a week is usually something that can be easily planned and adjusted for body type.

Once the meals are planned, write up a shopping list that contains all the needed ingredients. If you shop consistently at one store, plan the shopping list to follow the floor plan of the store with stops at the produce, bakery and frozen food departments last. You will notice that with a *Kids in Balance* eating style, most of your shopping will be around the outside perimeter of the store, with only the occasional foray into the middle aisle sections for items such as olive oil, salsa, herbal tea and natural peanut butter. The snack, cookie and cereal aisles will be visited only on rare, Sometimes Foods occasions.

Keep meals simple and enlist help for all the vegetable chopping! Roasted and sautéed meats or tasty legumes, hearty salads and steamed vegetables will be on the menu most evenings. That does not mean, however, that you cannot travel the world with changes in seasonings and style of cooking. Curries, stir-fries and stews from a variety of cultures all fit within the *KIB* eating plan.

And, if you have a bad day with some poor choices or lack of energy to prepare things the way you would like for your family, give yourself some grace. This is a lifestyle choice, not a quick fix. Get up the next day and have a family chat about getting back on track. Then, once you have your family to the place it should be health wise, if you aim for eating well at least 80% of the time, most bodies will still respond quite fine and love you mightily!

NOTE: 1) Capitalized/bolded ingredients are found as complete recipes elsewhere in the recipe section. 2) Some recipes contain an ingredient or two that should be omitted during days 8-21 of **Find Your BALANCE** and will be identified accordingly. 3) While most of the recipes can be used as is or adapted for days 8-21 of **Find Your BALANCE** a few need to be avoided completely until your child has completed *KIB*'s first phase. These recipes are marked with a **(B)** to remind you to wait to serve that recipe until your child is in **Build Your BALANCE**.

Appetizers and Snacks

Mini Florentine Turkey Cups   **(Makes 24)**

12 smaller-size slices turkey breast deli meat
1-10 ounce [225g] package frozen spinach, cooked, drained and finely chopped
2 eggs, preferably free range
2 tablespoons green onion, finely chopped
2 cloves garlic, minced (2 teaspoons)
¼ cup cheese [30g], preferably organic; shredded
1 tablespoon Parmesan cheese, grated

Preheat oven to 350°F [180°C]. Stir together all ingredients except turkey breast slices. Cut turkey slices in half and place one half in each of 24 lightly greased mini muffin pan cups, folding turkey slice as needed to fit muffin cup like a crust. Fill each cup with approximately 1½ teaspoons of spinach mixture. Bake Florentine cups in oven for 15 minutes or until heated through. Serve warm.

Trail Mix

A snack classic; never leave home without it!

raw nuts (i.e. almonds, pecans, walnuts, Valencia peanuts, hickory, macadamia and pine nuts)
raw seeds (i.e. pumpkin, sunflower, hemp, chia, salba, flax)
dried fruit (i.e. apricots, chopped; mission figs, chopped; prunes, chopped; raisins; unsweetened or lightly sweetened cranberries)
Optional: ½ teaspoon coconut oil or olive oil, pinch of sea salt and good quality chocolate chips

Preheat oven to 175°F [80°C]. Toss an assortment of nuts and seeds together (with the oil and sea salt if desired) and spread in one layer on a baking sheet. Bake nuts and seeds for 10-20 minutes. Cool and add in a variety of the listed dried fruits in a ratio of 3:1, nuts/seeds: fruit. For a Sometimes Foods occasion, add a small amount of chocolate chips.

(B) if including chocolate chips and/or dried fruits other than cranberries.

NOTE: Some people have trouble tolerating nuts. For those with allergies to certain nuts, those varieties will need to be omitted from any *KIB* recipes that contain them. For those, however, that simply have trouble digesting nuts, soaking nuts for 4-8 hours before eating raw or roasting can often rectify the situation. Soaking reduces nuts' naturally occurring but potentially problematic substances (i.e. enzyme inhibitors, phytic acid), enhances the availability of nutrients and enables the nuts to be more easily digested.

Spring Vegetable Platter

Veggie intake doesn't get any simpler or more kid-friendly than this!

snap peas
carrot sticks
radishes, halved
cucumber sticks
red pepper strips
zucchini [courgette] slices
celery sticks
cauliflower flowerettes
broccoli flowerettes

Wash and slice vegetables. Serve with **RANCH DRESSING** (p. 133).

Hot Artichoke Dip   (Serves 6)

This is a family favourite. For additional color and flavour add ½ cup of diced red pepper.

1 can (14 oz) [400g] artichoke hearts, drained and chopped
1 cup [250ml] **SIMPLE BLENDER MAYONNAISE** (p. 132) **or** good quality store bought mayonnaise (i.e. natural ingredients, low sugar content)
1 tablespoon green onion, minced
1 tablespoon red onion, minced
2 tablespoons parsley, finely chopped
2 cloves garlic, minced (2 teaspoons)
½ teaspoon lemon juice
Optional: ½ cup [50g] Parmesan cheese, grated

Preheat oven to 350°F [180°C]. Combine all ingredients and place in a shallow, ovenproof dish. Bake dip for 15-20 minutes until heated through and light golden color. Serve hot with vegetable dippers or, in **Build Your BALANCE**, in addition to vegetable dippers, serve with good quality crackers (i.e. whole grains, no refined sugar).

NOTE: For a flavour shift with a little more zip, substitute ½ cup [125ml] mayonnaise and ½ cup [125ml] plain yogurt, preferably organic, for the cup of mayonnaise.

Guacamole Pâté with Fresh Salsa   (Serves 12)

I love the elegant look of this pâté—almost as much as I love the smooth, yet bold flavour!

4 teaspoons [1½ packages-7g each] gelatin **or** use agar-agar per package directions
¼ cup [60ml] cold water
2 avocados, peeled and pitted
1 cup [250ml] full fat yogurt **or** sour cream, preferably organic
½ cup [125ml] **SIMPLE BLENDER MAYONNAISE or** good quality store bought mayonnaise (i.e. natural ingredients, low sugar content)
juice of 1 lemon (¼ cup) [60ml]
¼ teaspoon sea salt
¼ teaspoon pepper
⅛ teaspoon cayenne
2 cloves garlic, minced (2 teaspoons)
¼ cup [15g] cilantro, chopped
1 small tomato, finely chopped
1 small jalapeno pepper, seeded and finely chopped
2 green onions, finely chopped

Fresh Salsa

1 tomato, chopped
1 red pepper, seeded and chopped
1 jalapeno pepper, seeded and chopped
1 small red onion, minced
1 clove garlic, minced (1 teaspoon)
⅓ cup [20g] cilantro, chopped

In small saucepan, sprinkle gelatin over cold water and let stand for 1 minute. Heat gently over low heat for 2-3 minutes or until dissolved. In food processor, puree avocados, yogurt, mayonnaise, lemon juice, salt, pepper, cayenne and garlic until smooth. Blend in dissolved gelatin. Stir in cilantro, tomato, jalapeno pepper and green onions. Line 8 x 4 inch [20 x 10 cm] loaf pan with plastic wrap. Spoon in avocado mixture and cover with plastic wrap. Refrigerate for 3 hours or until set (can be refrigerated overnight).

For **Fresh Salsa**, combine all ingredients. Unmould pâté onto serving plate. Serve in slices with a spoonful of salsa spread down center of each slice.

Adapted from *The Canadian Living Christmas Book* by Elizabeth Baird and Anna Hobbs.

Roasted Red Pepper Boats   (Serves 4)

This recipe is a hit with the senses. The delicious aroma of fresh basil and olive oil will make your mouth water, while the brilliant colour combination of red, green and white entertain the eye. Substitute peppers of any colour in the summer when produce is at its freshest; stick to the recipe colour combination for a perfect Christmas appetizer.

2 large red peppers, each cut length-wise into 8 strips
1 tablespoon extra virgin olive oil
16 fresh basil leaves
½ cup [75g] feta cheese, preferably organic; crumbled

Preheat oven to 450°F [230°C]. Put red pepper into a mixing bowl; drizzle with olive oil and toss so oil lightly coats both sides of pepper strips. Spread peppers onto a baking sheet (preferably one with sides). Tear basil leaves to fit the bottom of each pepper chunk. Once each pepper is topped with a basil leaf, carefully top basil leaf with crumbled feta cheese. Roast on top rack until edges of pepper strips start to darken slightly.

For extra crunch, shorten baking time.

Spicy Hot Wings   (Serves 4)

28 chicken wings, cleaned and split
1 cup [250ml] hot sauce
1 cup [250ml] spicy salsa
½ cup [125ml] tamari **or** Kikkoman, naturally aged soy sauce
2 tablespoons granulated onion
2 tablespoons granulated garlic
2 tablespoons crushed red pepper flakes
1 teaspoon cayenne

Preheat oven to 300°F [150°C]. Place wings in single layer in a baking pan. Combine sauce ingredients. Reserve ¾ cup [200ml] of the sauce and pour remaining sauce over wings; bake for one hour. Remove wings and place on rack over a parchment paper-lined cookie sheet. Return chicken to oven and bake for 20 more minutes until chicken has a dry appearance. Baste chicken with some of the reserved sauce and continue baking. Baste wings 2-4 more times, at 5-minute intervals. Repeated basting increases the spiciness of the chicken. (As does doubling the salsa, like my son, Matt, does!)

Wings can also be marinated overnight in sauce prior to baking. Be sure to reserve ¾ cup [200ml] of sauce for basting before using remaining sauce for marinating wings.

Beans, Rice and Grains

Nut Barley Casserole (B) (Serves 8)

1 tablespoon coconut oil
1 medium yellow onion **and** 4 green onions, chopped
4 cloves garlic, minced (4 teaspoons)
2 carrots, finely diced
1½ cups [300g] pot barley
½ teaspoon each sea salt **and** pepper
4½ cups [1.1 litres] vegetable **or** chicken stock, homemade (p. 169) **or** good quality brand such as Imagine (i.e. natural ingredients, no MSG, no refined sugar)
2 tablespoons cilantro **or** parsley, minced
¾ cup [60g] slivered almonds, toasted

Preheat oven to 350°F [180°C]. On stovetop, in ovenproof casserole dish, sauté onions, garlic and carrots in coconut oil. When softened, stir in barley, salt and pepper; stir until well coated with oil. Add 2½ cups [600ml] of stock. Cover and bake for 30 minutes. Stir in cilantro and remaining 2 cups [500ml] stock. Sprinkle with almonds; bake 45 minutes until liquid is absorbed and barley done.

Fried Rice with Vegetables (B) (Serves 4)

3 tablespoons coconut oil, divided
1 cup [100g] carrots, thinly sliced
1 cup [100g] broccoli, in flowerettes
1 cup [100g] peas
1 cup [100g] snap peas, shredded
2 cups [60g] Swiss chard, shredded
¼ cup each parsley [15g], minced **and** green onion [40g], sliced thinly
2 cups [200g] brown rice, cooked and cooled
¼ teaspoon cayenne
4 tablespoons tamari **or** Kikkoman, naturally aged soy sauce
juice of 1 medium lemon (¼ cup) [60ml]
2 tablespoons water

Heat 1 tablespoon oil in wok over med-high heat. Stir-fry carrots for 1 minute; add broccoli, peas, snap peas and Swiss chard and stir-fry until vegetables are tender crisp. Add water to prevent sticking. Remove vegetables from wok. Heat remaining oil in wok. Add green onions and parsley and sauté for 1 minute. Add rice, tamari, cayenne, lemon juice and water; stir until heated through. Return vegetables to wok; stir until heated. Sprinkle with additional chopped parsley and serve.

Curried Rice (B)   (Serves 8)

If your family is just beginning a taste adventure with curry, start with 1 teaspoon of the paste.

3 cups [550g] brown basmati rice
1 tablespoon Patak's Madras curry paste
2 cans (14 oz) [400ml] unsweetened, coconut milk
2 cups [150g] unsweetened shredded coconut
1 large onion, diced
1½ tablespoons coconut oil, divided

Measure coconut milk and add 2½ cups [625ml] of water to make six cups [1.5 litres] liquid. Bring liquid to a boil, add rice and cook per package directions. While rice is cooking, dice onion and sauté in 1 tablespoon coconut oil. Remove onion from pan and set aside. Add remaining ½ tablespoon oil to pan and sauté coconut until lightly browned. When the rice is cooked, stir in onion, coconut and curry paste.

NOTE: If your family prefers spicier foods, add up to an additional tablespoon of curry paste.

Adapted from a recipe by Sandy Montgomery.

Sautéed Chickpeas   (Serves 2)

An easy protein-rich lunch addition!

1 can (19 oz) [540ml] chickpeas, drained
¼ cup [40g] red onion, slivered
1 red pepper, cut into strips
1 clove of garlic, minced (1 teaspoon)
1 tablespoon coconut oil
3 basil leaves, chopped (approximately 1 tablespoon)
¼ teaspoon pepper

Preheat large frying pan on medium heat. Heat coconut oil; add red onion and sauté until soft (approximately 4 minutes). Add red pepper and garlic and cook for 3 more minutes. Stir in chickpeas, cover and cook for a few minutes more. Remove from heat and stir in basil. Top with pepper.

NOTE: You can lightly toss mixed salad greens with **VINAIGRETTE** (p. 159) and serve the warmed chickpeas right on top of the greens. The slightly wilted lettuce leaves make a lovely change and provide a nice combination of warm and cold flavours.

Vegetarian Chili with Avocado Salsa (Serves 4)

2 teaspoons coconut oil
1 onion, chopped
1 red bell pepper, chopped
1 can (19 oz) [540ml] black, pinto **or** Romano beans, rinsed and drained
1 can (19 oz) [540ml] diced tomatoes
4 cups [1 litre] vegetable stock, homemade (p. 169) **or** good quality brand such as Imagine
(i.e. natural ingredients, no MSG, no refined sugar)
1 can (4 oz) [114ml] green chili peppers, chopped
2 teaspoons chili powder
2 cloves garlic, minced (2 teaspoons)
1 teaspoon cumin
1 teaspoon dried oregano
½ cup [125ml] sour cream, preferably organic
1 lime, quartered
2 tablespoons fresh cilantro, chopped

Avocado Salsa

1 medium avocado, peeled, pitted and finely chopped
1 small tomato, finely chopped
1 small green pepper, finely chopped
¼ red onion, finely chopped
2 cloves garlic, minced (2 teaspoons)
1 tablespoon fresh cilantro, chopped
juice of one lime (2 tablespoons)
¼ teaspoon cumin
¼ teaspoon pepper

Heat the oil in a 6-quart pot over medium heat. Add the onion and bell pepper and cook, stirring frequently, for 3 minutes. Add the beans, tomatoes (with juice), stock, chili peppers, chili powder, garlic, cumin, and oregano. Simmer for 20 minutes. Top individual bowls of chili with avocado salsa, a dollop of sour cream and a sprinkle of cilantro. Serve lime wedges on the side for those that like a squeeze of lime juice in their chili.

For **Avocado Salsa**, in a mixing bowl, combine the avocado, tomato, green pepper, onion, garlic, cilantro, lime juice, cumin and pepper. Lightly toss. Let stand for 30 minutes.

Adapted from *The South Beach Diet Cookbook* by Dr. Arthur Agatston MD.

Vegetable Chili (Serves 6)

A quick and easy rainy day supper, you can also put the ingredients together in a crock-pot. Leave it on low heat for the day and arrive home to an amazing aroma and taste that the whole family will enjoy.

2 tablespoons coconut oil
2 onions, chopped
3 carrots, diced
2 stalks celery, diced
3 cloves garlic, minced (3 teaspoons)
1 tablespoon cumin
2 teaspoons dried oregano
2 teaspoons natural seasoning salt (i.e. without MSG or sugar; brands such as Herbamare **or** Spike)
1 teaspoon dried basil
1 teaspoon dried marjoram
½ teaspoon cayenne
2 cups [325g] corn (omit during days 8-21 of **Find Your BALANCE**)
6 cups [1.5 litres] cooked pinto beans, drained (bean liquid reserved)
3 cups [750ml] reserved bean liquid (if not enough bean liquid remains, top up with water to make three cups or 750ml)
4 cups [1 litre] tomato puree **or** vegetable stock, homemade (p. 169) **or** good quality brand such as Imagine (i.e. natural ingredients, no MSG, no refined sugar)
1 zucchini [courgette], in ½ inch [1 cm] chunks

Mash two cups [500ml] of the pinto beans and set aside.

In a large saucepan heat oil. Add onions, carrots, celery, garlic, and seasonings and sauté, stirring constantly. When vegetables are well coated with oil, add corn, pinto beans (whole and mashed), tomato puree, bean liquid and zucchini. Bring chili to a boil, reduce heat and simmer covered for 30-45 minutes. Stir occasionally.

If a thicker chili is preferred, remove lid and simmer for an additional 10 minutes.

NOTE: For Protein Body Types, for either Vegetable Chili or Vegetarian Chili with Avocado Salsa (p. 128), add browned ground beef, bison, turkey or lamb.

Roasted Chickpeas   **(Makes 2 cups/425g)**

This recipe provides a handy portable protein for busy days. It can be used as an eat-alone snack, or can top a salad to make a complete meal. Missing popcorn on movie night? Have a small bowl of these with some veggies and dip.

1 can (19 oz) [540ml] chickpeas, drained, rinsed and patted dry
1 tablespoon coconut oil
¼ teaspoon garlic powder
¼ teaspoon onion powder
2 tablespoons Parmesan cheese, grated

Preheat oven to 350°F [180°C]. Choose a baking sheet with sides and line with parchment paper. In a mixing bowl, combine all the ingredients and toss until the chickpeas are evenly coated.

Spread chickpeas onto the baking sheet and bake for 60 to 75 minutes, or until the chickpeas are crisp (they will darken). Stir occasionally to promote even cooking. For extra nip, you can add a pinch of paprika or cayenne.

NOTE: These will disappear quickly, so you may want to double up and make two batches while you are at it. Bag them up into snack-sized portions (½ cup/105g) for easy lunch packing.

Mark's Hummus   **(Makes 2¾ cups/600g)**

1 tablespoon tahini (sesame seed paste)
¼ cup [60ml] extra virgin olive oil
2 cloves garlic, minced (2 teaspoons)
2 cups chickpeas [400g], cooked
¼ cup [60ml] reserved chickpea liquid
1 tablespoon lemon juice
1 teaspoon dried cumin
¼ cup parsley [15g]

Place tahini, olive oil, and garlic in food processor. Process for 1-2 minutes. Add chickpeas, reserved chickpea cooking liquid and lemon juice; process until chickpeas are smooth. Add cumin and parsley, process for an additional minute.

Serve with vegetable dippers or, in **Build Your BALANCE**, in addition to vegetable dippers, serve with good quality pita bread or crackers (i.e. whole grains, no refined sugar).

Quick Breads

Carrot-Apricot Muffins (B) (Makes 24)

2½ cups [250g] carrot, grated
⅔ cup [160ml] honey
3½ cups [875ml] apple juice **or** a combination of apple juice and coconut milk
⅔ cup [160ml] olive, safflower **or** coconut oil
3 cups each whole wheat flour [450g] **and** unbleached white flour [420g]
1½ cups [230g] rolled oats
½ cup [100g] millet **or** a combination of flax **and** chia seeds [65g]
1 tablespoon aluminum-free baking powder
2 teaspoons baking soda
1 cup [130g] dried apricots, diced

Preheat oven to 400°F [200°C]. Beat together grated carrots, honey, apple juice and oil. In a separate bowl combine flours, rolled oats, millet, baking powder and baking soda. Add wet mixture to dry ingredients. Mix just until combined; stir in apricots. Fill muffin cups ¾ full. Bake 17-20 minutes until golden.

Orange Scones with Almonds and Dates (B) (Makes 12)

1 cup each whole wheat flour [150g] **and** unbleached white flour [140g]
1 tablespoon lemon juice
1 tablespoon grated orange rind
½ teaspoon stevia powder
½ teaspoon baking soda
½ cup [90g] dates, chopped
⅓ cup coconut oil [75ml] **or** butter [75g], preferably organic **or** Better Butter (see **NOTE** below)
½ cup [125ml] coconut milk **or** plain yogurt, preferably organic
½ cup [125ml] orange juice
¼ cup [20g] raw almonds, chopped

Preheat oven to 425°F [220°C]. Grease baking sheet or line with parchment paper. Combine dry ingredients, lemon juice, orange rind, stevia and baking soda in food processor. Cut in oil until mixture resembles coarse crumbs. Add coconut milk, orange juice, dates and almonds and process just until moistened. On sheet of wax paper, pat dough to 1½ inch [4 cm] thickness and, using 2 inch [5 cm] diameter cookie cutters, cut out 12 scones. Bake for 11 minutes and serve immediately.

NOTE: Better Butter is equal parts butter and olive oil, blended and stored in the refrigerator.

Dressings and Sauces

Simple Blender Mayonnaise (Makes 1½ cups/375 ml)

This classic is easy to make and is the foundation for a variety of sauces and dressings.

2 eggs, preferably free range
1 tablespoon lemon juice
1 tablespoon apple cider vinegar
½ teaspoon sea salt
¼ teaspoon dry mustard **or** ½-1 tablespoon Dijon mustard to taste
1 cup [250ml] olive oil

Put the eggs, lemon juice, apple cider vinegar, salt, pepper and mustard into blender (or food processor). Cover and blend at medium speed for 5 seconds.

With blender running at low speed, add the oil very slowly (i.e. with the thinnest stream you can make). For best results the oil should hit the egg mixture about ½ way between the sides of the blender and the vortex in the middle and should take about two minutes to add. Blend until no more oil remains on the surface of the mayonnaise.

Keeps covered in the refrigerator for up to 1 week.

Lime Butter (Makes 1¼ cups/300ml)

¾ cup [170g] butter, preferably organic
¼ cup [60ml] coconut oil
2 tablespoons parsley, minced
juice of one lime (2 tablespoons)
1 teaspoon honey (omit during days 8-21 of **Find Your BALANCE**)
1 teaspoon pepper
1 teaspoon chili powder
½ teaspoon cumin
½ teaspoon sea salt
1 small clove garlic, minced (½ teaspoon)

Process butter, oil, parsley and lime juice in blender or food processor until smooth.

Add remaining ingredients and serve on corn on the cob. Lime butter is also a tasty topping for grilled or steamed vegetables.

Tofu Sour Cream   (Makes 1½ cups/375ml)

¼ cup [60ml] olive oil
juice of 1 lemon (¼ cup) [60ml]
2 tablespoons water
¼ teaspoon natural seasoning salt (i.e. without MSG or sugar; brands such as Herbamare)
1 can (4 oz) [114ml] jalapeno peppers, diced
8 ounces [250g] soft tofu, in chunks

Put the olive oil, lemon juice, water, seasoning salt and jalapeno peppers into blender (or food processor). Cover and blend at medium speed for 30 seconds. With blender running at medium speed, add tofu. Process until smooth. Refrigerate 1-2 hours to meld flavors. Keeps covered in the refrigerator for 3-4 days.

OPTION: if your family likes things a little less spicy, substitute pinches of coriander and cumin and a bit of lime juice for the jalapeno peppers.

Ranch Dressing Seasoning Mix and Dressing   (Makes 3½ cups/350ml)

This dry seasoning mix is great to keep on hand for making fresh vegetable dips!

15 whole grain crackers, blended until powdered (omit during days 8-21 of **Find Your BALANCE**)
2 cups [10g] dry parsley flakes
1 cup [60g] dry minced onion
½ cup [30g] garlic powder
¼ cup [15g] onion powder
2 tablespoons dried dill weed
1 teaspoon sea salt
½ teaspoon pepper

Blend crackers (if using), parsley, minced onions and dill weed. Stir into remaining dry ingredients. Store mixture in container with tight fitting lid for up to 1 year. Makes 40-1 tablespoon servings.

Ranch Dressing

1 heaping tablespoon **RANCH DRESSING MIX**
1 cup [250ml] **SIMPLE BLENDER MAYONNAISE** (p. 132) **or** good store bought mayonnaise
1 cup [250ml] buttermilk **or** yogurt **or** sour cream (**or** combination of all three), preferably organic

To make **Ranch Dressing**, stir all ingredients together well in a bowl. Serve as a dip with assorted fresh vegetables or as a creamy salad dressing. Keeps covered in the refrigerator for 3-4 days.

Spring Salad Dressing

(Makes 1¼ cups/300ml)

⅓ cup [80ml] each apple cider vinegar **and** olive oil
1 tablespoon lemon juice
2 green onions, chopped
2 teaspoons each fresh dill **and** parsley, chopped
¼ teaspoon natural seasoning salt (i.e. without MSG or sugar; brands such as Herbamare)

Combine all ingredients, except olive oil, in a blender or food processor. Blend on high for 15 seconds until parsley is well chopped. With blender running on low speed, slowly add olive oil to mixture. Serve immediately on your favourite green salad or refrigerate for up to three days.

Barbeque Sauce

(Makes 1 cup/250ml)

1 can (8 oz) [250ml] tomato sauce
2 tablespoons apple cider vinegar
1 teaspoon Worcestershire sauce
1 teaspoon mustard powder
1 teaspoon dried parsley
¼ teaspoon stevia powder **or** ½ teaspoon molasses (days 8-21 of **Find Your BALANCE** use stevia)
¼ teaspoon each sea salt **and** pepper
2 cloves garlic, minced (2 teaspoons)
5 drops Tabasco

In a resealable container, combine all ingredients. Keeps covered in the refrigerator for 1 week.

Ketchup

(Makes 1 cup/250ml)

1 can (8 oz) [250ml] tomato sauce
¾ cup [200ml] tomato paste
½ teaspoon stevia powder
2 teaspoons onion powder
2 teaspoons tamari **or** Kikkoman, naturally-aged soy sauce
½ teaspoon each ground cloves **and** allspice
1½ tablespoons apple cider vinegar
1 bay leaf

In a large pot over medium heat, combine all ingredients. Simmer for 5 minutes. Remove bay leaf. Refrigerate until serving. Keeps covered in the refrigerator for 1 week.

Eggs

Scrambled Eggs Supreme

(Serves 2)

Or as our kids call it, "Eggs the Way You Like It!"

4 large eggs, preferably free range
1 tablespoon green onion, minced
⅛ teaspoon sea salt
½ tablespoon coconut oil **or** butter, preferably organic
pepper to taste

ADD-ONS

1 tablespoon red onion, diced
2 tablespoons red pepper, diced
1 turkey pepperoni stick, sliced
¼ cup [25g] mushrooms, sliced
¼ cup [25g] tomatoes, diced
1 breakfast-sized beef, bison **or** lamb sausage, cooked and diced or crumbled

Heat oil in skillet over medium high heat. Choose desired **ADD-ON** ingredients and sauté in pan until softened and heated through. While **ADD-ON** ingredients cook, beat the eggs in a medium bowl with green onion and salt. Add the egg mixture to the **ADD-ON** ingredients in the pan and cook, stirring frequently until eggs reach desired doneness. Add pepper before serving.

Spinach-Zucchini Frittata   (Serves 3)

1 tablespoon coconut oil **or** butter, preferably organic; divided
1 cup [30g] fresh spinach, chopped **or** frozen spinach, thawed and drained
¾ cup each zucchini [courgette] [75g] **and** onion [120g], chopped
1 tablespoon fresh oregano **or** ½ teaspoon dried oregano
1 tablespoon basil **or** ½ teaspoon dried basil
6 large eggs, preferably free range
¼ teaspoon each sea salt **and** pepper
1 cup [150g] goat feta

Preheat broiler. In medium ovenproof skillet, melt ½ tablespoon coconut oil over medium-high heat. Add the spinach, zucchini and onions and sauté until vegetables are softened, about 3 minutes. In medium bowl, combine cooked vegetables and herbs and feta.

In separate bowl, beat eggs with salt and pepper. In skillet, melt remaining coconut oil over medium-high heat and then pour egg mixture into skillet. Cook, gently stirring until bottom of egg starts to set. Continue cooking (without stirring) until top is just slightly runny. Remove from heat and sprinkle with vegetable mixture. Place frittata under broiler for 2 minutes until golden colored.

Tex-Mex Breakfast Eggs   (Serves 4)

½ tablespoon coconut oil **or** butter, preferably organic
½ cup each green pepper [50g] **and** onion [80g], chopped
8 large eggs, preferably free range, slightly beaten
¾ cup [200ml] salsa, divided
2 cloves garlic, minced (2 teaspoons)
½ teaspoon cumin
1½ cups [170g] cheddar cheese, preferably organic, divided
1 avocado, diced
Optional: 8 corn taco shells, heated

Melt coconut oil or butter in skillet. Add pepper and onions to skillet and cook until just tender. Stir in eggs, ¼ cup [60ml] of the salsa, garlic and cumin. Cook over medium heat, stirring gently, until eggs reach desired doneness. Remove from heat and stir in 1 cup [115g] of the cheddar cheese. Divide egg mixture on 4 plates and top each mixture with ¼ of the diced avocado, 2 tablespoons of remaining salsa and 2 tablespoons of remaining cheese.

NOTE: After **Find Your BALANCE**, eggs can be served in taco shells. Divide egg mixture between shells; top each with ⅛ of the diced avocado, 1 tablespoon of salsa and 1 tablespoon of cheese.

Asparagus Omelet (Serves 2)

If your child is not yet a fan of asparagus, this omelet works well with a wide variety of vegetables. Try additional peppers or grated zucchini and carrots.

1½ tablespoons coconut oil **or** butter, preferably organic; divided
½ cup [80g] onions, diced
2 cups [200g] asparagus, in 1 inch [2 cm] pieces
½ cup [50g] red peppers, chopped
½ cup [50g] mushrooms, chopped
2 tablespoons cilantro **or** basil, minced
⅛ teaspoon sea salt
⅛ teaspoon pepper
4 large eggs, preferably free range
2 tablespoons water

Sauté vegetables in ½ tablespoon coconut oil until tender crisp, starting with the onions and peppers and adding the mushrooms and asparagus after a couple of minutes. Stir in the cilantro, salt and pepper.

While vegetables are cooking, beat the eggs with the water and salt. When vegetables are done, transfer to a medium sized bowl. In skillet, over medium-high heat, melt another ½ tablespoon coconut oil in skillet. When oil is hot, add half the egg mixture and cook until almost at desired doneness, lifting the edges of the omelet with a spatula while tilting the skillet and letting the uncooked portion run to the bottom. Spoon half the vegetable mixture onto one half of the omelet, fold other half of omelet over the filling and slide onto serving plate.

Melt the last ½ tablespoon of coconut oil in the skillet and repeat the procedure for the second omelet. Serve immediately.

Fish

Cod Teriyaki   (Serves 4)

4 cod fillets, 4-6 ounces [100-175g] each
½ cup [125ml] tamari **or** Kikkoman, naturally-aged soy sauce
juice of 1 lemon (¼ cup) [60ml]
3 tablespoons freshly grated ginger

Combine marinade ingredients and pour over fish fillets. Refrigerate for several hours. Discard marinade. Preheat BBQ to high heat and then grill fish for 6-8 minutes per side until cod reaches an internal temperature of 160°F [71°C] or flakes easily with a fork. Fish can also be broiled in oven for the same amount of time.

NOTE: Fresh ginger can be stored in a freezer bag for up to 3 months. Simply cut off a frozen piece, as you need it. The flavour will still be fresh and lively.

Succulent Grilled Salmon   (Serves 4)

1 large salmon fillet, with skin on, about 1½ pounds [700g]
¼ teaspoon hot pepper sauce
juice of one lemon (¼ cup) [60ml]
2 tablespoons cilantro, minced
2 cloves of garlic, minced (2 teaspoons)
pepper to taste

Preheat BBQ to high heat. Place salmon on grill, skin side down (if skinless, lay salmon on a piece of parchment paper-lined aluminum foil on the grill and poke foil with a knife to allow juices to escape). Combine remaining ingredients to make sauce. Baste salmon generously with the sauce and grill until salmon is partially cooked (6-8 minutes). Turn salmon, leaving skin or foil on the grill and baste with additional sauce. Grill until salmon is cooked (3-5 minutes) and flakes easily with a fork.

After days 8-21 of **Find Your BALANCE**, this salmon is delectable with a homemade mango salsa: dice one large mango and combine with two tablespoons of diced red onion, 1 tablespoon of minced cilantro, 1 tablespoon diced jalapeno and 1 tablespoon of lime juice.

NOTE: Cilantro stays fresh for up to two weeks in your fridge if you place it in a tall container filled with about 2 inches [5 cm] of water. Cover cilantro loosely with a plastic bag (i.e. a clear plastic produce bag) and change water every other day.

Barbequed Salmon Baste

(Serves 4)

4 salmon fillets, 4-6 ounces [100-175g] each
⅔ cup [165ml] **SIMPLE BLENDER MAYONNAISE** (p. 132)
⅓ cup [80ml] coconut oil **or** [75g] butter, preferably organic; melted
1 tablespoon honey **or** ⅛ teaspoon stevia powder (use stevia days 8-21 of **Find Your BALANCE**)
1 tablespoon apple cider vinegar
2 teaspoons dill, chopped
juice of ½ lemon (1½ tablespoons)

Preheat BBQ to high heat. Place salmon on grill, skin side down (if skinless, lay salmon on a piece of parchment paper-lined aluminum foil on the grill and poke foil with a knife to allow juices to escape). Combine remaining ingredients to make sauce. Baste salmon generously with the sauce and grill until salmon is partially cooked (6-8 minutes). Turn salmon, leaving skin or foil on the grill and baste with additional sauce. Grill until salmon is cooked (3-5 minutes) and flakes easily with a fork. Discard any remaining basting sauce. If you would like to serve sauce on the side, make extra sauce, beyond what you make for basting, to serve with salmon.

Adapted from a recipe by Sandy Montgomery.

Grilled Flounder with Rosemary

(Serves 4)

Lovely topped with capers.

4 flounder fillets, 4-6 ounces [100-175g] each
2 teaspoons extra virgin olive oil
2 teaspoons lemon juice
¼ teaspoon sea salt
¼ teaspoon pepper
2 cloves garlic, minced (2 teaspoons)
2 teaspoons fresh rosemary leaves, minced **or** 1 tsp dried rosemary leaves, crushed

Combine the olive oil, lemon juice, salt, pepper, garlic and rosemary in a bowl. Brush the mixture onto the fish. Marinate flounder in refrigerator for 2-4 hours or cook immediately.

Preheat BBQ to high heat. Place flounder on BBQ and grill for 6-8 minutes per side until fish reaches an internal temperature of 160°F [71°C] or flakes easily with a fork. To broil in the oven, brush the rack of a broiler pan with olive oil and arrange the fish on it. Broil 4 inches [9 cm] from the heat. Same cooking time applies.

Grilled Salmon with Lime and Cilantro   (Serves 4)

4 salmon fillets, 4-6 ounces [100-175g] each
1 tablespoon grated lime rind
juice of one lime (2 tablespoons)
2 tablespoons olive oil
¼ cup [15g] cilantro, finely chopped
2 tablespoons green onion, chopped
2 tablespoons cilantro, chopped
Optional garnish: lime wedges

Combine grated rind and juice of lime with olive oil and ¼ cup [15g] of cilantro. Pour marinade over salmon and refrigerate for several hours.

Preheat BBQ to high heat. Remove fillets from marinade and discard marinade. Grill fillets for 6-8 minutes per side, until fish flakes easily with a fork. Remove to serving platter and sprinkle with green onion and cilantro. Garnish with lime wedges and serve immediately.

Asian Flounder with Vegetables   (Serves 4)

4 flounder fillets, 4-6 ounces [100-175g] each
¼ cup [60ml] olive oil
2 tablespoons tamari **or** Kikkoman, naturally-aged soy sauce
juice of 1 lemon (¼ cup) [60ml]
2 tablespoons parsley, chopped
1 teaspoon freshly grated ginger
1 green onion, chopped
1½ cups [150g] carrots, julienned (omit during days 8-21 of **Find Your BALANCE**)
1½ cups [150g] cauliflower, in flowerettes
1½ cups [150g] green beans, in 1 inch [2 cm] pieces
Optional garnish: parsley, chopped

To make marinade, combine oil, tamari soy sauce, lemon juice, parsley, ginger and green onion. Reserve 2 tablespoons of marinade for vegetables. Marinate flounder fillets in remaining marinade for 30 minutes. Remove fillets from marinade (discard marinade) and bake (20 minutes at 350°F/180°C) or grill (6-8 minutes a side on high heat) until opaque and flesh flakes easily with a fork. While fish cooks, heat reserved marinade in a large skillet or wok. Add vegetables and stir-fry for 5- 7 minutes until tender crisp. If mixture becomes too dry, add 1-2 tablespoons water.

Place flounder on a platter. Surround with vegetables and garnish with parsley.

Meat

Curried Beef or Lamb with Vegetables   (Serves 6)

*A mild tasting curry that, in **Build Your BALANCE** and beyond, is wonderful over brown basmati rice.*

2 pounds [900g] of lamb **or** beef stewing meat
3 tablespoons coconut oil
1½ tablespoons freshly grated ginger
4 cloves garlic, minced (4 teaspoons)
2 onions, sliced
2 carrots, chopped (omit during days 8-21 of **Find Your BALANCE**)
3 cups [300g] vegetables (i.e. cauliflower, zucchini, green beans), chopped
⅔ cup [160ml] apple cider vinegar
1 cup [250ml] water

Paste

1½ tablespoons ground coriander
1 teaspoons ground cardamom
1 teaspoons ground cloves
½ teaspoon cayenne
⅓ cup [80ml] apple cider vinegar

Mix **Paste** ingredients together and set aside.

Over medium heat, in large saucepan, heat 2 tablespoons of the coconut oil. Sauté ginger root and garlic in oil for 2 minutes, stirring constantly. Add and brown stewing meat. Remove meat and set aside.

Melt remaining tablespoon of coconut oil in pan. Add and sauté onions until golden. Add paste and cook onions an additional 5 minutes, stirring constantly. If mixture becomes too dry, add one or two additional teaspoons of vinegar or water.

Return meat to pan and add the ⅔ cup [160ml] apple cider vinegar and water. Bring mixture to a boil, cover and simmer for 15 minutes. Add carrots and other chopped vegetables; return to a boil. Then reduce heat and simmer for an additional hour until meat is tender.

Bison Lettuce Wraps with Peanut Sauce (Serves 4)

¼ cup [60ml] **SIMPLE BLENDER MAYONNAISE** (p. 132)
¼ cup [60ml] 100% Valencia peanut butter
2 tablespoons water
2 tablespoons unpasteurized honey (omit during days 8-21 of **Find Your BALANCE**)
2 tablespoons tamari **or** Kikkoman, naturally-aged soy sauce
1 tablespoon freshly grated ginger **or** 1 teaspoon ground dried ginger
4 bison steaks, 3–4 ounces [115-150g] each, grilled or broiled
1 cup [100g] carrots, grated
¼ cup [40g] green onion, chopped
16 large lettuce leaves

For sauce, stir **SIMPLE BLENDER MAYONNAISE**, peanut butter, water, tamari, honey and ginger in small saucepan on medium heat just until heated through. Do not overcook. Slice bison steaks. Divide meat and vegetables into quarters and arrange on four serving plates. Diners roll a portion of their meat, carrots and green onion up in a lettuce leaf, dip the wrap in peanut sauce and enjoy!

NOTE: The wraps also work well with beef, lamb or chicken.

Best Barbecued Burgers (Serves 4)

1 pound [450g] lean ground beef
⅓ cup [80ml] tomato sauce
¼ teaspoon sea salt
¼ teaspoon pepper
2 cloves of garlic, minced (2 teaspoons)
½ cup [15g] basil leaves, torn into small pieces
¼ teaspoon hot pepper sauce
½ cup [50g] Parmesan cheese, grated

Mix all ingredients together in a bowl, adding the Parmesan cheese last. Form into patties and barbeque on grill until done, basting with **BARBECUE SAUCE** (p. 134).

Wash whole pieces of red or green lettuce leaves and serve separately for wrapping burgers. Condiments can include homemade ketchup, red onion, unsweetened dill pickles, mustard, tomato and cheese.

NOTE: In **Build Your BALANCE**, if desired substitute ½ cup wheat germ for Parmesan cheese and, in any phase, double the recipe and save leftovers for a tasty and simple lunch the next day.

Roast Bison or Beef with Harvest Vegetables (Serves 6)

If making the recipe with bison, remember it is generally very lean meat and can be easy to overcook. Reduce cooking time slightly and watch closely near the end of the time.

3 pound [1.35kg] sirloin tip **or** similar quality cut bison **or** beef roast
2 teaspoons apple cider vinegar
1 teaspoon lemon juice
1 teaspoon natural seasoning salt (i.e. without MSG or sugar; brands such as Herbamare)
1 teaspoon pepper

Harvest Vegetables

1 red onion, in wedges
1 red pepper, in large chunks
1 yellow pepper, in large chunks
1 zucchini [courgette], in thick slices
1 leek, in thick slices
2 carrots, cut in 1 inch [2 cm] pieces (omit during days 8-21 of **Find Your BALANCE**)
2 celery stalks, cut in 1 inch [2 cm] pieces
1 tablespoon olive oil
1 tablespoon lemon juice
2 tablespoons apple cider **or** balsamic vinegar

Preheat oven to 450°F [230°C]. Place roast, fat side up, in a roasting pan. Combine apple cider vinegar, lemon juice, natural seasoning salt and pepper and drizzle over roast. Cook uncovered for ½ hour. Reduce heat to 300°F [150°C], cover roast, and cook for another 1¼ - 1¾ hours for medium doneness.

About an hour before the roast is done, wash and prepare onion, peppers, zucchini, leek, carrots and celery for **Harvest Vegetables**, and place in another ovenproof dish. Toss vegetables with olive oil and lemon juice and bake covered for 45 minutes. Just before serving, toss hot vegetables with balsamic vinegar and enjoy with roast.

NOTE: To make a full meal salad, serve vegetables and slices of roasted meat atop mixed salad greens. Top with your favourite *Kids in Balance* salad dressing.

Moroccan Beef Stew

(Serves 8)

Though simple enough to prepare for a family dinner, makes tasty and impressive company fare as well!

3 pounds [1.35kg] beef stewing meat
3 tablespoons coconut oil, divided
2 leeks, chopped **or** 1 cup [120g] pearl onions
5 cloves garlic, minced (5 teaspoons)
3 large carrots, chopped (substitute whole green beans during days 8-21 of **Find Your BALANCE**)
1 can (19 oz) [540ml] diced tomatoes
1 teaspoon cumin
1 teaspoon coriander
1 tablespoon freshly grated ginger
½ teaspoon sea salt
½ teaspoon pepper
¼ teaspoon cinnamon
fresh parsley, chopped
2 cups [500ml] beef stock, homemade (p. 169) **or** good quality brand such as Imagine (i.e. natural ingredients, no MSG, no refined sugar)
Optional garnish: fresh parsley, chopped

If using oven, pre-heat oven to 325°F [160°C]. In heavy saucepan, heat 1½ tablespoons of the oil over medium heat and brown beef, stirring often. Set beef aside.

Add remaining 1½ tablespoons oil to saucepan and sauté leek, garlic and carrots until softened, stirring often. Add tomatoes and seasoning, except parsley, and cook, stirring constantly, for one minute. Stir in stock and bring to a boil.

Cover pan and simmer for 3-3 ½ hours on stovetop until meat is tender. Alternatively bake in oven in covered, ovenproof pan for same amount of time.

Garnish with parsley and serve.

Adapted from *The Canadian Living Christmas Book* by Elizabeth Baird and Anna Hobbs.

Really Good Beef and Bean Chili   (Serves 4)

When appropriate for KIB phase and your child's body type, this chili tastes great served over a halved baked potato.

1 pound [450g] lean ground beef **or** bison
1 yellow onion, chopped
1 cup [160g] corn (omit during days 8-21 of **Find Your BALANCE**)
1 cup [100g] diced carrot (omit during days 8-21 of **Find Your BALANCE**)
1 cup [100g] celery, chopped
1 large red pepper, chopped
3 cloves garlic, minced (3 teaspoons)
1 tablespoon chili powder
1 tablespoon apple cider vinegar
½ teaspoon ground thyme
¼ teaspoon sea salt
¼ teaspoon pepper
¼ teaspoon cumin
¼ teaspoon ground oregano
½ teaspoon hot pepper sauce
1 can (28 oz) [796ml] diced tomatoes
1 can (19 oz) [540ml] red kidney beans **or** black beans, drained and rinsed
1 can (4 oz) [114ml] chopped green chili peppers
2 tablespoons fresh parsley, minced

In large pot, sauté beef over medium heat, breaking up with spoon, until no longer pink, about 5 minutes. Drain off fat. Add onion, celery, (carrots in **Build Your BALANCE**), pepper, garlic, chili powder, thyme, salt, pepper, cumin, oregano and hot pepper sauce to pan; fry, stirring occasionally, until onion is softened, about 4 minutes. Stir in tomatoes and beans (and corn in **Build Your BALANCE**); bring to boil. Reduce heat and simmer until thickened, about 20 minutes. Just before serving, stir in parsley.

Adapted from *Canadian Living Magazine: Winter 2006.*

Rockin' Roast Beef

(Serves 4)

A good old standby, given an updated name by my daughter, Rachel!

1 beef chuck pot roast (2.5–3 pounds) [1.1-1.35kg]
1 tablespoon extra virgin olive oil
¾ cup [200ml] low-sodium beef stock, homemade (p. 169) **or** good quality brand such as Imagine (i.e. natural ingredients, no MSG, no refined sugar)
½ cup [125ml] dry red wine (not during **Find Your BALANCE**), tomato juice **or** tomato sauce
1 tablespoon Worcestershire sauce
½ cup [15g] basil, torn or chopped in small pieces
3 cloves of garlic, minced (3 teaspoons)
¼ teaspoon hot pepper sauce
¼ teaspoon pepper
Optional: 1 large onion, in chunks

Preheat large frying pan on medium heat. Heat olive oil. Remove excess fat from roast and brown all sides in hot oil. To make sauce, combine remaining ingredients, except for the pepper, in a small mixing bowl. Place roast in an oven roasting pan and carefully pour sauce over the roast so that some of the basil and garlic remain atop the roast. Top with pepper. Bake, covered, in a 325°F [160°C] oven for 1 hour and 45 minutes. If using onion, place in the pan around the roast for the last 45 minutes to add extra aroma and flavour.

Serve sliced on a platter, ladling cooking juices over top for a delectable, moist finish.

After **Find Your BALANCE**, add a couple of chopped sweet potatoes or small red potatoes to the pan after the roast has cooked for about 50 minutes.

NOTE: When serving leftovers in a lunch, you can cube the cooked meat and soak it overnight in the juices. Then, skewer the meat and send as tender shish kabobs for lunch.

Homemade Shake and Bake Pork (B)   (Serves 4)

1 cup [115g] whole grain cracker crumbs (crush about 15 crackers in a Ziploc bag)
¼ cup [25g] Parmesan cheese, grated
¼ cup [20g] almonds, finely chopped (use food processor or coffee bean grinder)
1 clove garlic, minced (1 teaspoon)
2 tablespoons parsley, chopped
¼ teaspoon thyme
sea salt **and** pepper to taste
⅓ cup [80ml] extra virgin olive oil
4 boneless pork rib chops
Optional garnish: ½ cup [80g] green onions, chopped

Preheat oven to 400°F [200°C]. In a medium-sized mixing bowl, combine cracker crumbs, cheese, almonds, parsley, garlic, thyme, salt and pepper. Pour oil into a shallow dish (i.e. a small rectangular glass cooking pan). Coat the pork chops first in oil and then with the crumb mixture. Place the coated pork in a shallow baking dish. Pat mixture into any gaps on the pork for a nice even coating. Cover and bake for 35–40 minutes or until a meat thermometer inserted in the center of the chop reads 170°F [77°C] and juices run clear. Do not turn during cooking. Top with green onion.

NOTE: This recipe also works well with boneless, skinless chicken breasts. Cook for approximately 25–30 minutes.

Pork Tenderloin with Lime Marinade   (Serves 6)

½ cup [125ml] vegetable stock, homemade (p. 169) **or** good quality brand such as Imagine
juice of 3 limes (½ cup) [125ml]
2 cloves of garlic, minced (2 teaspoons)
1 teaspoon chili powder
½ teaspoon cumin
¼ teaspoon each ground coriander, sea salt, **and** pepper
2 pork tenderloins, about 1 pound [450g] each

In a large mixing bowl, combine all ingredients except the pork. Before marinade comes in contact with meat, reserve ⅓ cup [80ml] in sealed container to use later for basting. Add tenderloins, turning to coat. Cover and marinate in fridge for 4–24 hours. Preheat BBQ to medium heat. Remove pork from marinade and discard marinade. Place pork on oiled grill, brushing with reserved marinade. Grill with closed lid. Turn pork occasionally, until meat thermometer reads 170°F [77°C]. This will take approximately 18-20 minutes. Transfer finished tenderloin to a cutting board, tenting with foil for 5-10 minutes before slicing into serving portions.

No-Dough Pizza with Homestyle Pizza Sauce (Serves 2)

This meal can serve as either a snack or the protein-rich portion of a lunch. Kids love feeling like they are eating pizza again!

2 thick slices of ham, chicken **or** turkey (**or** good quality, thickly cut deli meat)
1 green onion, chopped
¼ cup [25g] red pepper, diced
⅓ cup [30g] part skim mozzarella cheese, preferably organic; shredded

Homestyle Pizza Sauce

3 tablespoons tomato sauce
pinch garlic powder **or** 1 clove of garlic, minced (1 teaspoon)
1 teaspoon fresh basil, chopped **or** ¼ teaspoon dried basil
⅛ teaspoon dried oregano
sea salt **and** pepper to taste

Place oven rack 4-6 inches [9-13 cm] from broiler. Preheat oven to broil.

Put both slices of ham, chicken or turkey on a baking sheet, in a single layer; set aside.

To make **Homestyle Pizza Sauce**, in a small bowl, mix together tomato sauce, basil, oregano, salt and pepper. Spread pizza sauce evenly on both slices of meat. Sprinkle with green onions and red pepper, and top with shredded cheese.

Broil for 3-5 minutes or until cheese has reached a golden brown. Remove pizza, cool slightly and serve. Give your child the pizza cutter to cut it into bite-sized pieces—much more fun than a fork and knife!

Roast Loin of Pork with Herbed Filling (Serves 5)

You will need kitchen twine & wooden picks for this recipe.

1 boneless center loin pork roast, about 2 pounds [900g]
¾ teaspoon sea salt
½ teaspoon pepper
1 tablespoon extra virgin olive oil
Optional garnish: fresh sage leaves and rosemary sprigs

Herbed Filling

2 tablespoons parsley, chopped
1½ tablespoons sage **or** thyme leaves, chopped
1 tablespoon rosemary, chopped
3 cloves garlic, minced (3 teaspoons)
3 tablespoons extra virgin olive oil
2 teaspoons Dijon mustard
¼ sea salt
¼ teaspoon ground black pepper

To make **Herbed Filling, i**n a small bowl, combine filling ingredients.

Preheat the oven to 350°F [180°C]. Butterfly the pork loin. (Position the pork lengthwise on a cutting board. Cut in the center of the roast lengthwise, going only halfway down. Spread this cut open and cut sideways in either direction to open the roast up to a long rectangular shape.) Using a kitchen mallet, pound the loin to an even thickness, just enough that you will be able to roll it up neatly. Spread the filling evenly across loin, leaving a ¼ inch [.5 cm] border along the edges.

Roll the loin up to wrap the filling. Using kitchen twine, tie the loin every 2-3 inches [5-7 cm] to hold its shape. Rub the loin with the oil and sprinkle with the remaining salt and pepper. Place the loin in a small roasting pan and position on the center rack of the oven. Roast for 1 hour or until a thermometer inserted in meat registers 160°F [71°C] and the juices run clear.

Let stand for 10 minutes before carving. To prevent slices from unrolling, skewer the roast every ¼-½ inch [.5-1 cm] with wooden picks along the edge where the roll ends. Slice crosswise between the wooden picks and ties. Remove kitchen twine before serving.

Tuscan Layered Lasagna

(Serves 5)

A favourite of my daughter, Rebekah, this delicious dish is easily individualized to handle any KIB phase.

Tomato Layer

3 cups [600g] tomatoes, chopped (cherry **or** grape tomato halves **or** large tomatoes diced)
2 tablespoons extra virgin olive oil
2 cloves garlic, minced (2 teaspoons)
1 teaspoon dried basil (**or** 2 tablespoons fresh basil, chopped)
½ teaspoon sea salt

Ricotta Layer

drizzle of extra virgin olive oil
2 cups [400-450g] ricotta cheese, preferably organic
3 tablespoons basil pesto sauce, homemade **or** good quality store bought (i.e. natural ingredients, no or low sugar content)

Meat Sauce

1½ pounds [700g] lean ground bison **or** beef
1 large red **or** yellow onion, diced
2 cloves garlic, minced (2 teaspoons)
1 tablespoon chili powder
2 teaspoons paprika
¼ teaspoon nutmeg
¼ teaspoon pepper
1 can (19 oz) [540ml] diced tomatoes, including juice

8 lasagna noodles (B); for **Find Your BALANCE**, substitute spinach **or** zucchini slices

Preheat oven to 375°F [190°C]. Have ready two baking dishes, one 8 x 8 inches [20 x 20 cm] and one 9 x 13 inches [23 x 32 cm]. Combine **Tomato Layer** ingredients and spoon mixture, in a single layer, into the small baking dish. For **Ricotta Layer**, drizzle olive oil in the large baking dish, and spread ricotta cheese evenly in dish. On top of ricotta, spread pesto sauce. Place the pans of tomatoes and ricotta cheese in the oven to bake for about 20 minutes while completing the next steps.

Bring a large pot of salted water to boil. Meantime, to make **Meat Sauce**, drizzle olive oil into a large sauté pan and heat at medium high heat. Sauté meat, onion, garlic and meat sauce spices until meat is browned. Add canned tomatoes and simmer for 10-15 minutes.

To boiling salted water add lasagna noodles and cook, per package directions, until done. If using spinach or zucchini, lightly steam vegetables until done (i.e. spinach is bright green and slightly wilted; zucchini is heated through and softened). When tomatoes and ricotta have baked for 20 minutes, broil them for 2-3 minutes until lightly browned at edges and remove from oven. Cut ricotta into 12 equal sized pieces.

To build lasagnas, begin by spooning a small amount of juice from tomatoes onto individual serving plates. Fold lasagna noodle in ½ and place on juice, top with a small amount of meat sauce and a couple spoonfuls of roasted tomatoes, another lasagna noodle, three pieces of ricotta, more meat sauce and a couple more spoonfuls of tomatoes and their juice. Serve immediately.

Adapted from *House and Home* magazine online.

Meatballs on a Stick   (Serves 4)

These meatballs make yummy snacks or appetizers!

1 cup [60g] parsley, finely chopped and lightly packed
2 green onions, chopped
1 clove garlic, minced (1 teaspoon)
½ teaspoon dried oregano
½ teaspoon sea salt
¼ teaspoon pepper
1 large egg, preferably free range
1 pound [450g] lean ground beef
tzatziki sauce, homemade **or** good quality store bought (i.e. natural ingredients, no or low sugar)

4 whole wheat pita breads (omit during days 8-21 of **Find Your BALANCE**)

In a food processor, mix the parsley, green onion, garlic, oregano, salt and pepper. Blend in egg and transfer mixture to a large bowl. Add beef and mix well. Shape into oval meatballs, almost sausage-like in shape, and thread lengthwise onto metal or pre-soaked wooden skewers.

Preheat BBQ to medium-high or oven to broil. Grill the skewers on barbeque or under oven broiler. On the barbeque, cook with the lid closed, turning meatballs once after about 6 minutes. They should only take about 12 minutes. In the oven, cook for 7-10 minutes. In either case, meat thermometer should read 160°F [71°C].

If using pita bread, during the last minute or two of cooking, toss the pitas onto the grill or into the oven, until they have reached desired crispness (it does not take long, so keep watch). Cut each pita into 6 pie-shapes wedges and serve with tzatziki sauce for dipping. For days 8-21 of **Find Your BALANCE**, use tzatziki sauce (without sugar) if desired, but take a pass on the pita bread.

Poultry

Chicken Lasagna-Style   (Serves 4)

1 cup [250g] ricotta cheese, preferably organic
½ teaspoon dried oregano
¼ teaspoon sea salt
¼ teaspoon pepper
4 boneless, skinless chicken breast halves, 4-6 ounces [100-175g] each
½ teaspoon garlic powder
2 tablespoons extra virgin olive oil
1 cup [250ml] tomato sauce
4 slices mozzarella cheese, preferably organic

Preheat over to 350°F [180°C]. In a small bowl or a blender, combine the ricotta with the oregano, salt and pepper. Rub the chicken with the garlic powder. Heat the oil in a large skillet over medium-high heat. Add the chicken and cook for 10 minutes per side. Place the chicken breasts, side by side, in a large baking dish. Spoon ¼ cup [63g] of the cheese mixture and ¼ cup [60ml] tomato sauce onto each chicken breast. Top each chicken breast with 1 slice of mozzarella. Bake for 15–20 minutes, or until a thermometer inserted in the thickest part of the breast registers 170°F and the juices run clear. For a golden brown top, set the oven to broil for the last 3 minutes.

Barbecued Garlic Chicken   (Serves 6)

3-4 pounds [1.3-1.7kg] of chicken thighs
½ cup [120ml] tamari **or** Kikkoman, naturally-aged soy sauce
¼ cup [60ml] olive oil **or** coconut oil
juice of 1 lemon (¼ cup) [60ml]
2 tablespoons apple cider vinegar
2 tablespoons green onion, chopped
2 teaspoons ginger, grated
1 teaspoon honey (omit during days 8-21 of **Find Your BALANCE**)
3 cloves garlic, minced (3 teaspoons)

Combine marinade ingredients and pour over chicken thighs. Refrigerate for several hours. Preheat BBQ to medium-high heat. Remove chicken from marinade (discard marinade). Barbecue chicken for 35 minutes, turning after 15-20 minutes.

NOTE: Chicken can also be oven-baked at 400°F [200°C] for 30-35 minutes.

Chicken Souvlaki   (Serves 2)

2 boneless, skinless chicken breasts, 4-6 ounces [100-175g] each
juice of 1 lemon (¼ cup) [60ml]
3 tablespoons olive oil **or** coconut oil
1 teaspoon dried oregano
2 cloves garlic, minced (2 teaspoons)
8 mushrooms
1 leek, cut in chunks
1 medium zucchini [courgette] cut in 1 inch [2 cm] chunks
8 cherry tomatoes

Combine lemon juice, olive oil, oregano and garlic for marinade. Reserve 2 tablespoons of marinade for basting. Cut chicken into 1½ inch [3 cm] chunks and marinate in lemon juice/oil mixture in refrigerator for 1-2 hours.

Remove chicken from marinade and discard marinade. Arrange chicken alternately with vegetables on 4-6 skewers. Pre-heat BBQ to medium-high. Brush souvlaki skewers with reserved marinade and grill for 5-7 minutes per side.

Simple Chicken Curry   (Serves 6)

4 boneless chicken breasts, 4-6 ounces [100-175g] each, in 1 inch [2 cm] pieces
2 tablespoon coconut oil
3 large carrots, in ½ inch [1 cm] pieces (omit during days 8-21 of **Find Your BALANCE**)
½ medium cauliflower, in flowerettes
1 red pepper, in 1 inch [1 cm] pieces
1 large red onion, in 1 inch [1 cm] pieces
1½ cup [150g] green beans, fresh **or** frozen
2 cans (14 oz) [400g] unsweetened coconut milk
1-2 tablespoons good quality prepared Madras curry paste (i.e. Patak's)

Heat 1 tablespoon coconut oil in skillet and sauté chicken pieces until cooked through and no pink remains. Remove chicken from pan and add remaining tablespoon of oil to pan.

Sauté carrots in heated oil for 2-3 minutes; add cauliflower, pepper, onion and green beans. When vegetables are heated through and softened but still tender-crisp, add chicken back to pan and stir in curry paste. When paste is well distributed, stir in coconut milk and cook until heated through.

NOTE: After **Find Your BALANCE**, curry can be served with brown basmati rice.

Mediterranean Grilled Chicken   (Serves 4)

A surprising combination of cinnamon and oregano flavours for a BBQ delight!

juice of 1 lemon (¼ cup) [60ml]
2 tablespoons extra virgin olive oil
2 tablespoons fresh oregano, chopped **or** 1 teaspoon dried oregano
½ teaspoon pepper
½ teaspoon cinnamon
½ teaspoon paprika
¼ teaspoon sea salt
4 boneless, skinless chicken breast halves, 4-6 ounces [100-175g] each

Combine all ingredients except the chicken in a small bowl and stir for marinade. Once well mixed, pour marinade into a large zip-lock plastic bag. Add chicken breasts and squeeze bag to evenly distribute marinade to coat chicken. Seal bag, removing excess air and store in the fridge for 30 minutes, flipping once halfway through.

Preheat BBQ to medium-low heat. Remove chicken from bag and discard marinade. Grill chicken on barbeque for 12–15 minutes or until chicken is cooked through (6–7 minutes per side).

Blackened Turkey Thighs   (Serves 6)

6 large turkey thighs, 4-6 ounces [100-175g] each **or** 12 small-medium chicken thighs, 2-4 ounces [50-90g] each
2 tablespoons paprika
1 teaspoon onion powder
1 teaspoon garlic powder
½ teaspoon white pepper
½ teaspoon black pepper
½ teaspoon sea salt
½ teaspoon dried thyme
½ teaspoon dried oregano
¼ teaspoon cayenne
Optional: coconut oil

Combine seasoning ingredients.

Coat turkey with spice mixture, drizzling meat with a small amount of coconut oil if mixture will not stick well. Grill turkey until cooked through and no pink remains.

Turkey Roll-Ups

(Serves 1)

A tasty treat!

2 whole green **or** red lettuce leaves
1 green onion, chopped
2 strips of red **or** yellow bell pepper
¼ teaspoon yellow **or** Dijon mustard
2 tablespoons good quality store bought mayonnaise (i.e. natural ingredients, low sugar content)
2 thin slices of good quality deli meat (turkey, chicken, ham)
Optional: unsweetened dill pickle and tomato slices

Wash and pat dry the lettuce leaves, cutting off any stiff parts at the bottom (this makes it easier to roll). Spread leaves out sideways for filling. Combine mustard and mayonnaise in a small bowl. Using spatula or a kitchen basting brush, spread half of mixture on each lettuce leaf, up to ¼ inch [.5 cm] from edges. Layer each leaf with 1 or 2 slices of deli meat, and top with 1 strip of bell pepper, and pickle and tomato slices if using. Sprinkle with green onion. Roll width-wise and enjoy a tasty, filling treat.

NOTE: If you like cilantro, add ½ cup chopped cilantro to mayonnaise and serve on the roll-ups. It takes a little longer to prepare this version, but it tastes sensational.

Asian Chicken Drumsticks

(Serves 4)

16 chicken drumsticks
½ cup [125ml] tamari **or** Kikkoman, naturally-aged soy sauce
½ cup [125ml] apple juice (see **NOTE** for **Find Your BALANCE**)
2 tablespoons honey **or** unrefined cane sugar (see **NOTE** for **Find Your BALANCE**)
3 cloves garlic, minced (3 teaspoons)
1 tablespoon paprika
1 tablespoon cayenne

Preheat oven to 350°F [180°C]. Combine sauce ingredients and pour over chicken. Bake for 30-40 minutes until chicken is cooked through and no pink remains.

NOTE: For days 8-21 of **Find Your BALANCE**, prepare sauce ingredients without apple juice and honey or unrefined cane sugar. Substitute ½ cup water and a pinch of stevia.

Salads

Caesar Salad I   (Serves 2)

1 small head romaine lettuce, torn into bite-sized pieces

Dressing

1 clove garlic, minced (1 teaspoon)
1 teaspoon Dijon mustard
juice of 1 lemon (¼ cup) [60ml]
¼ cup [60ml] extra virgin olive oil
¼ teaspoon sea salt

In a wooden salad bowl, whisk the following **Dressing** ingredients: garlic, Dijon mustard, lemon juice and salt. Gradually whisk in olive oil. Add lettuce to bowl and toss. Serve immediately.

Caesar Salad II   (Serves 4)

1 head romaine, torn into bite-sized pieces
1 small handful of Parmesan cheese, grated (roughly 4 teaspoons)

Dressing

½ cup [120ml] extra virgin olive oil **or** walnut oil
1 egg, preferably free range
1 teaspoon each lemon juice **and** water
½ tablespoon Worcestershire sauce
sea salt **and** pepper to taste
pinch dry mustard
3 cloves of garlic, minced (3 teaspoons)

Twenty minutes before you wish to serve the salad, combine the following **Dressing** ingredients in blender and mix to combine: oil and egg. Add lemon juice and water and mix again. Add salt, pepper, dry mustard and garlic. Mix for 1 minute in blender. Place dressing in refrigerator for 15 minutes.

Combine romaine and Parmesan together in a salad bowl. Add dressing and toss to coat.

Grated Vegetable Salad (Serves 4)

2 cups [200g] carrots, grated
3 cups [300g] cabbage, grated
1 cup [100g] green pepper, grated
½ red onion, grated

Dressing

¼ cup [60ml] each olive oil **and** apple cider vinegar
juice of 1 lemon (¼ cup) [60ml]
1 tablespoon fresh dill, chopped **or** 1 teaspoon dried dill
1 teaspoon natural seasoning salt (i.e. without MSG or sugar; brands such as Herbamare)

Combine vegetables in bowl. Whisk together **Dressing** ingredients and mix into vegetables. Chill salad for at least 30 minutes. Serve.

Bean Salad with Vegetable Relish (Serves 2)

2 cups [200g] green beans
2 cups [200g] each red leaf lettuce **and** butter lettuce
1 cup [250g] cooked, chilled mixed beans (i.e. chickpea, pinto, lima)
½ medium red onion, thinly sliced

Vegetable Relish

¼ cup each, parsley [15g], radishes [25g] **and** spinach [10g], finely chopped
½ green pepper, finely chopped
1 carrot, grated
1 green onion, minced
⅓ cup [80ml] each apple cider vinegar **and** olive oil
¼ teaspoon sea salt

Lightly steam green beans until tender crisp. Plunge beans into cold water, drain, cut in half and refrigerate. At serving time, tear lettuces into bite-sized pieces and divide between two plates. Arrange mixed beans, red onion slices and green beans on lettuce. Combine **Vegetable Relish** ingredients, cover and refrigerate. Spoon relish over beans and garnish with whole radishes. Serve.

Asian Cabbage Salad   (Serves 6)

1 medium head Chinese cabbage, shredded
½ bunch green onions, finely chopped
⅓ cup each raw almonds [25g], slivered **and** sesame seeds [50g]
1 tablespoons coconut oil

Dressing

1 tablespoon tamari **or** Kikkoman, naturally-aged soy sauce
¼ cup [60ml] honey (omit during days 8-21 of **Find Your BALANCE**) **or** pinch of stevia powder to taste
¼ cup [60ml] each olive oil **and** apple cider vinegar

Mix cabbage and green onions together. (Mixture can be refrigerated overnight.) Heat coconut oil in a skillet and sauté almonds and sesame seeds until light brown. Remove from heat. When nuts and seeds are cool, stir into cabbage mixture. To make **Dressing**, in a small covered container, shake together the soy sauce, honey or stevia powder, olive oil and vinegar until well combined. Toss salad with dressing just before serving.

Lemony Spinach and Artichoke Salad   (Serves 4)

A blissful ensemble of flavours, and easy to make too!

1 large bunch spinach
1 can (14 oz) [400g] artichoke hearts packed in water
⅓ cup [30g] Parmesan cheese, grated

Dressing

¼ cup [60ml] extra virgin olive oil
1 clove of garlic, minced (1 teaspoon)
2 teaspoons lemon peel, freshly grated
1 tablespoon lemon juice
2 tablespoons red wine vinegar

Wash and dry spinach. Cut off long stems and rip gently into bite-size pieces. Place in salad bowl, cover and refrigerate until ready to use. Drain and quarter artichoke hearts. To make **Dressing**, combine all the dressing ingredients in blender or in a jar. Process or shake to combine, and refrigerate for at least 15 minutes before using. Just before serving, top spinach leaves with artichoke chunks and Parmesan. Drizzle with dressing and toss gently to carefully coat salad.

Green Salad with Radishes (Serves 2)

3 cups [300g] assorted lettuces, torn into bite-sized pieces
1 cup [130g] asparagus, in 1 inch [2 cm] pieces, lightly steamed and chilled
½ cup [65g] cucumber, diced
½ cup [50g] radishes, quartered

Vinaigrette

3 tablespoons olive oil
juice of 1 lemon (¼ cup) [60ml] **or** ¼ cup [60ml] balsamic vinegar
½ teaspoon Dijon mustard
¼ teaspoon sea salt
1 clove garlic, minced (1 teaspoon)

Place lettuces in salad bowl. Add remaining vegetables. Whisk or shake together **Vinaigrette** ingredients. Gently toss salad with dressing.

Flavours of Summer Salad (Serves 4)

8 cups [800g] mixed organic greens
½ red onion, slivered
⅓ cup [25g] pecans, roasted
1 red bell pepper, sliced into strips
1 ripe avocado, peeled, pitted and cubed

Combine ingredients and toss lightly with homemade (p. 159) or good quality store bought vinaigrette (i.e. natural ingredients, no or low sugar content) for a delicious and textured salad. Add black beans and/or chunks of cooked chicken breast to make a satisfying meal.

Marinated Beet Salad (B) (Serves 3)

6 medium beets
2 tablespoons each olive oil **and** lemon juice
¼ cup [40g] green onions, sliced
1 teaspoon tarragon

Steam beets until tender crisp. Under cold running water, slip skin from beets and then thinly slice. Marinate beet slices for a least one hour in remaining ingredients. Serve.

Tomato and Bocconcini Salad   (Serves 2)

For a handy buffet version of this salad, thread the stacks on a skewer as we did for the wedding reception of my son, Sam, and his lovely wife, Megan. The "salad on a stick" was a very fun and tasty hit!

12 medium cherry **or** grape tomatoes
3 mini balls of bocconcini, sliced into coin shapes **or** ¾ cup [85g] mozzarella, in large cubes
¼ cup [60ml] each extra virgin olive oil **and** balsamic vinegar
2 tablespoons capers
½ small red onion, slivered
½ red pepper, cut into strips
4 cups [400g] mixed greens, **or** romaine lettuce torn into bite-size pieces

Preheat large frying pan on medium heat. Heat olive oil; add balsamic vinegar, salt and pepper. Add red onion and sauté until soft, about 4 minutes. Add red pepper and cook for 3 more minutes. Stir in capers, cover and cook for 2 minutes more. Remove from heat. Pour complete mixture into a mixing bowl and put in fridge to cool.

Halve small tomatoes and combine with cheese in a salad bowl. Once the dressing has cooled, add the salad greens to the tomatoes and cheese. Add onion and pepper mix and toss to coat the salad.

OPTIONS:

MOZZA-CUKE STACKS: For a kid-friendly version of these flavours, stack thin slices of mozzarella on top of cucumber rounds. Arrange four stacks on a small dessert or salad plate and dot balsamic vinegar or **BALSAMIC REDUCTION** (see **TIP**) on top and around the stacks. If desired, a fresh basil leaf can be inserted between the cucumber and the cheese for an extra burst of flavour.

TOMATO-BOCCONCINI STACKS: Place slices of tomato on a serving platter; drizzle each with a bit of extra virgin olive oil. Top each with a small fresh basil leaf and top with a round of bocconcini or mozzarella cheese. Dot plate and stacks with balsamic vinegar. Fresh, easy and yummy!

NOTE: If this is your first time trying bocconcini, note that it has a mild taste, and a spongy texture that absorbs flavours well.

TIP: Rather than purchase a bottled supply, make **BALSAMIC REDUCTION** easily at home. In a small saucepan, heat 1-2 cups [250-500ml] balsamic vinegar on medium-high heat, whisking constantly, until vinegar has thickened, and has reduced in volume by half. Reduction can also be made in a double boiler as this greatly reduces the chance of scorching. Store in squeeze bottle.

Full Meal Salads
(Serves 1)

2 cups [200g] leaf lettuce, spinach, romaine **or** mixed field greens, torn into bite-sized pieces
1 cup [about 100g] steamed cauliflower, broccoli, green beans **or** asparagus; **and** 1 cup [about 100g] raw cucumbers, red pepper strips, grated carrot, avocado, zucchini **or** tomatoes
½ cup [30g] parsley, cilantro, kale **or** bitter greens
½ cup raw nuts [40g] **or** canned black beans [50g] **or** leftover cooked beef, bison, lamb, salmon, chicken **or** turkey strips [80g]
2 tablespoons each extra virgin olive oil **and** organic apple cider vinegar **or** lemon juice
1 tablespoon fresh herbs (i.e. basil, chives, parsley), chopped

Toss greens, vegetables and nuts, beans or meat together on serving plate. Whisk together olive oil and vinegar or lemon juice with herbs. Drizzle dressing over salad and serve.

NOTE: If desired, substitute Feta or other cheese for a portion of the protein-rich ingredients.

Mediterranean Chicken Salad with Tahini Dressing
(Serves 2)

4 cups [400g] red leaf lettuce, torn into bite-sized pieces
2 cups [320g] cooked chicken, cooled and diced
2 cups [200g] broccoli flowerettes, lightly steamed and cooled
1 cup [30g] alfalfa sprouts
1 cup [130g] cucumber, in ½ inch [1 cm] chunks

Tahini Dressing

3 tablespoons tahini (sesame seed paste)
1 tablespoon grated lemon rind
juice of 1 lemon (¼ cup) [60ml]
1 tablespoon each green onion **and** parsley, chopped
¼ teaspoon sea salt
½ cup water
Optional garnish: parsley sprigs and thin slices of lemon

Make **Tahini Dressing** by combining tahini, lemon juice and rind, green onion, parsley and salt in a blender (or use a hand blender). Process ingredients on high for 45 seconds. Reduce blender speed to medium. Slowly add water and blend until dressing is thick and smooth. For salad, combine all ingredients in a large bowl and gently toss with dressing. Garnish with parsley sprigs and slices of lemon.

Stacked Summer Salad   (Serves 6)

1 red pepper, in strips
1 yellow pepper, in strips
3 medium tomatoes, diced **or** 1½ cups grape tomatoes
2 cups [200g] broccoli flowerettes, lightly steamed
1 cup [100g] baby carrots, lightly steamed (serve raw during days 8-21 of **Find Your BALANCE**)
1½ cups [240g] red onion, diced
1 cup [200g] chickpeas **or** navy beans, cooked
1 cup [200g] Greek olives
1 cup [150g] Feta cheese, preferably organic
¾ cup [200ml] extra virgin olive oil
½ cup [125ml] apple cider vinegar
2 teaspoons Dijon mustard
2 teaspoons parsley, minced
2 teaspoons cilantro, minced
2 cloves garlic, minced (2 teaspoons)
1 teaspoon each sea salt **and** pepper

In large glass salad bowl, layer pepper strips, broccoli, carrots, onion, beans, olives, Feta and tomatoes.

Blend together olive oil, vinegar, Dijon mustard, parley, cilantro, garlic, salt and pepper. Pour dressing over salad and refrigerate for 24 hours.

Chicken Caesar   (Serves 4)

4 boneless chicken breasts, 4-6 ounces [100-175g] each, in 1 inch [2 cm] pieces
1 tablespoon coconut oil
1 large head of Romaine lettuce, torn into bite-sized pieces
CEASAR DRESSING I or II (p. 156)
¼ cup [25g] fresh grated Parmesan cheese
homemade whole grain croutons (i.e. 1 inch/2 cm whole grain bread cubes sautéed in butter and minced garlic until crisp; omit during days 8-21 of **Find Your BALANCE**)

Heat 1 tablespoon coconut oil and sauté chicken pieces until cooked through and no pink remains. Place salad greens in large bowl. Add chicken and toss with **CAESAR DRESSING** (see **CAESAR SALAD I or II** recipe) and Parmesan cheese.

If using croutons, add and serve immediately.

Make-Your-Own Taco Salad   (Serves 4)

This is a wonderfully easy meal for family members to personalize for their own body type.

1 pound [450g] lean ground beef, bison **or** lamb
1 cup [200g] pinto **or** kidney beans, cooked and cooled **or** substitute canned beans
2 medium carrots, grated
1 seedless cucumber, diced
½ medium red onion, diced
1 can (8 oz) [250ml] ripe, black olives, sliced
8 cups [800g] salad greens (romaine, red leaf, endive), torn into bite-sized pieces
TOFU SOUR CREAM (p. 133)
Taco seasoning to taste (i.e. chili powder, cumin, coriander, cayenne)
Corn chips **and** salsa (omit corn chips during days 8-21 of **Find Your BALANCE**)

Brown ground meat, adding favorite taco seasonings. Set meat aside.

Place salad greens into a large bowl. Gently toss in grated carrots and cucumber. Place meat, red onion, olives, beans, corn chips, salsa and **TOFU SOUR CREAM** each in individual serving bowls to make a salad bar.

Divide lettuce/vegetable mixture on serving plates and allow each diner to create their own taco salad. Enjoy!

NOTE: If desired, substitute Salsa Dressing (mix together equal parts salsa with yogurt) for the **TOFU SOUR CREAM**.

Chef's Salad (Serves 4)

A kid-friendly salad that adults love as well!

5 ounces [150g] good quality turkey **or** ham deli meat, thinly sliced
6 cups [600g] mixed lettuce greens, torn into bite-sized pieces
1 cup [130g] cucumbers, thinly sliced
½ cup [50g] carrot, grated
4 hard-boiled eggs, preferably free range, cut into wedges
⅔ cup [65g] broccoli, in small flowerettes
½ cup [65g] cheddar **or** Swiss cheese, preferably organic; shredded

Dressing

⅓ cup [80ml] extra virgin olive oil
¼ cup [60ml] red wine vinegar
2 tablespoons green onions, chopped
1 tablespoon Dijon mustard
¼ teaspoon sea salt
¼ teaspoon pepper

Roll up turkey or ham slices and cut into thin strips. In a large salad bowl, combine meat, salad greens, cucumber, carrot and broccoli.

To make **Dressing**, in a jar or a mixing bowl, combine olive oil, red wine vinegar, green onions, Dijon mustard, salt and pepper. Shake in jar or whisk in bowl to combine. Store in fridge until ready to serve.

When serving time, pour dressing over top of salad and toss to evenly coat salad. Garnish with egg wedges and sprinkle with cheese.

Soups

Hearty Pea Soup   (Serves 8)

Nothing says "comfort food" like a bowl of this soup on a cold, rainy day!

1 onion, diced
2 tablespoons coconut oil **or** olive oil
1½ cups [300g] dried yellow split peas
1½ cups [300g] dried green split peas
½ cup [100g] dried navy beans
⅓ cup [65g] pot barley (omit during days 8-21 of **Find Your BALANCE**)
11 cups [2.75 litres] water
2 teaspoons sea salt
1 teaspoon dried basil
1 teaspoon dried marjoram
½ teaspoon dried tarragon
2 cups [200g] carrots, diced (omit during days 8-21 of **Find Your BALANCE**)
½ cup [30g] parsley, chopped

In a large soup pot sauté onion in coconut oil. When onion is soft, stir in split peas, navy beans, pot barley, water and seasonings. Bring soup to a boil and then reduce heat and simmer for 50 minutes. Add carrots and simmer for an additional 30-40 minutes. Ten minutes before serving, stir in parsley.

NOTE: For Protein Body Types add ½ inch [1 cm] chunks of cooked turkey kielbasa or bison sausage when adding in parsley.

Bean Soup with Cumin   (Serves 8)

2 cups [400g] dried black **or** pinto beans
12 cups [3 litres] vegetable stock, homemade (p. 169) **or** good quality brand such as Imagine (i.e. natural ingredients, no MSG, no refined sugar)
2 tablespoons coconut oil
1 large onion, chopped
3 cloves garlic, minced (3 teaspoons)
4 carrots, diced (omit during days 8-21 of **Find Your BALANCE**)
2 teaspoons cumin
½ teaspoon sea salt
Optional garnish: 2 green onions, sliced

Cover beans with cold water and let soak overnight. Drain beans and combine with vegetable stock. Bring soup to a boil and then reduce heat and simmer for 3 hours or until beans are very tender.

Heat oil in skillet and sauté onion and garlic until softened. Add carrots and stir and cook an additional 2-3 minutes. Add vegetable mixture and seasonings to beans. Simmer soup for an additional 30 minutes. Working in batches, puree soup in blender (or use hand blender). Return soup to pot and gently heat soup to serving temperature. Garnish with green onions.

Borscht (B)   (Serves 4)

6 cups [1.5 litres] water
2 cups [200g] beets, julienned
1 cup [100g] carrots, diced
¼ cup [15g] parsley, chopped
1 onion, diced
1 tablespoon coconut oil
2 cups [200g] cabbage, chopped
½ teaspoon sea salt

Bring beets and water to a boil. Reduce heat and simmer 15 minutes. While soup simmers, sauté carrots, parsley and onions in oil for 3-4 minutes, stirring constantly. Add sautéed vegetables, cabbage and salt to soup and let simmer for an additional 15-20 minutes. Serve.

NOTE: For Protein Body Types add strips of leftover roast beef or browned lamb sausage.

Sopa de Tortilla with Tex-Mex Onions   (Serves 6)

This soup is easy to double for a crowd and is a hit with even my non-soup-loving son, Joel.

10 cups [2.5 litres] water
2 large carrots, in ½ inch [1 cm] chunks (omit during days 8-21 of **Find Your BALANCE**)
1 large onion, chopped
3 stalks celery, chopped
3 cloves garlic, minced (3 teaspoons)
2 cups [200g] cauliflower, chopped
2 cups [325g] corn (omit during days 8-21 of **Find Your BALANCE**)
2 cups [200g] broccoli stalks, peeled and in ½ inch [1 cm] chunks
2 cups [200g] zucchini [courgette], in ½ inch [1 cm] chunks
6 tomatoes, chopped
¼ cup [10g] cilantro, chopped
1 teaspoon dried oregano
½ teaspoon cumin
½ teaspoon sea salt
½ teaspoon cayenne

Tex-Mex Onions

2 tablespoons olive oil **or** coconut oil
2 large onions, sliced
2 green chili peppers, diced
¼ cup [60ml] medium **or** hot salsa
Optional garnish: corn chips

In large soup pot, bring water to boil and add carrots, chopped onion, celery and garlic. Reduce heat and simmer covered, for 5 minutes. Add cauliflower, corn (if using) and broccoli stalks. Cover pot, return soup to a boil and simmer for 10 minutes. Add zucchini, tomatoes, cilantro, cumin, salt and cayenne. Return soup to boil, then reduce heat and simmer for 5 more minutes.

For **Tex-Mex Onions**, heat oil and then sauté onions and chili peppers for 3-4 minutes. Add salsa to skillet and continue sautéing until onion is wilted. Place a tablespoon of Tex-Mex Onions and ½ cup [15g] corn chips (if using) in bottom of each individual soup bowl. Ladle soup over onions and chips and serve immediately.

NOTE: For Protein Body Types add chunks of leftover barbecued chicken or browned ground beef meatballs.

Minestrone Soup   (Serves 10)

This soup makes a high-fibre, packed full of goodness, meal!

2 tablespoons extra virgin olive oil
1½ cups [240g] onion, chopped
2 cloves garlic, minced (2 teaspoons)
1 cup [100g] each celery **and** carrots, thinly sliced (omit carrots during days 8-21 of **Find Your BALANCE**)
1 cup [100g] green pepper, chopped
4 cups [400g] unpeeled zucchini [courgette], cubed
2 cups [200g] green beans, in 1 inch [2 cm] pieces
1 can (35 oz) [992g] Italian plum tomatoes, including juice
2 cups [500ml] chicken stock, homemade (p. 169) **or** good quality brand such as Imagine (i.e. natural ingredients, no MSG, no refined sugar), **or** water
handful of basil leaves, torn into pieces **or** 1 teaspoon dried basil
½ teaspoon dried oregano
sea salt **and** pepper to taste
1 can (19 oz) [540ml] chickpeas, drained
1 can (19 oz) [540ml] kidney beans **or** black beans, drained
3 cups [300g] cabbage, finely sliced
Optional garnish: fresh parsley, chopped

In a large pot, heat the oil. Add onion, garlic, celery, carrots, and green pepper. Sauté until the onion is tender (approx 4 minutes). Add zucchini, green beans, tomatoes, stock, basil, oregano, salt and pepper and mix gently. Cover and simmer slowly for 40 minutes, stirring occasionally.

Add the chickpeas, kidney or black beans and cabbage. Cover and simmer about 15 minutes longer, or until cabbage is tender, stirring once or twice.

The soup will be thick, like a stew. If you like a thinner soup, add more stock or water. Garnish lavishly with parsley before serving.

Adapted from *The Anti-Breast Cancer Diet Cookbook*.

Zuppa Toscana (Serves 4)

8 medium-sized spicy Italian sausages, preferably turkey
1 leek, finely chopped
1 medium-sized bunch of kale, chopped into small pieces
2 cups [200g] broccoli stalks, peeled and chopped
4 cups [1 litre] chicken stock, homemade (p. 169) **or** good quality brand such as Imagine
2 cups [500ml] cream, preferably organic
10 Yukon Gold potatoes, in ½ inch [1 cm] cubes (omit during days 8-21 of **Find Your BALANCE**)
1 teaspoon of dried pepper flakes

Squeeze sausage meat out of skins into a large saucepan. Brown on high heat. Add a bit of the chicken stock if the meat sticks to the bottom. When the meat is cooked add the rest of the stock, leek, broccoli stalks and pepper flakes (and potato is using). Turn the heat down to simmer. When the broccoli is cooked, add kale and cream. Turn the heat down to low so the cream won't curdle and heat thoroughly, about 15-20 minutes. Serve.

Adapted from a recipe by Sandy Montgomery.

Stock (Serves 8)

A simple start to so many good soups, stews and chilies.

3 pounds [1.3kg] of bones (i.e. beef, bison **or** lamb **or** chicken **or** turkey carcass)
3 carrots, in 1 inch [2 cm] pieces
2 medium yellow onions, in 1 inch [2 cm] pieces
2 stalks celery, in 1 inch [2 cm] pieces
4 cloves garlic
¼ cup [60ml] apple cider vinegar
1 small bunch parsley, coarsely chopped

Place all ingredients, except for the parsley, in a large stockpot. Cover ingredients with 12-14 cups [3-3.5 litres] of water, making sure water does not come within 1 inch [2 cm] of the top of the pot. Bring water to a boil, then lower heat and simmer stock for 3-6 hours. About 15-20 minutes before you finish cooking the stock, add parsley. Strain broth, discard bones and vegetables, and refrigerate stock until cool. Remove congealed fat that will collect on the top of the stock. Use stock within a day or two or, alternatively, freeze stock for later use.

NOTE: For vegetable broth, replace bones with a wide range of heartier vegetables (i.e. carrots, parsnips, kohlrabi, broccoli stalks) and with the parsley, add additional greens (i.e. kale).

Tomato Soup   (Serves 4)

Tomatoes are a great source of lycopene and vitamins C and A. That makes this timeless favourite a tasty way to up your family's phytochemical intake.

1 can (28 oz) [796ml] Italian crushed tomatoes
2 tablespoons extra virgin olive oil
1 large onion, chopped
3 cloves garlic, minced (3 teaspoons)
1½ tablespoons tomato paste
⅛ teaspoon stevia powder (to taste)
4 cups [1 litre] vegetable stock, homemade (p. 169) **or** good quality brand such as Imagine (i.e. natural ingredients, no MSG, no refined sugar)
handful basil leaves, torn into small pieces
sea salt **and** pepper to taste
Optional: zucchini, mushrooms and sweet bell peppers, and ½ cup [65g] shredded cheese

Over medium heat, heat oil in large pot. Add chopped onion to the pan and sprinkle garlic on top of the onion. Put lid on the pot and let cook for a couple of minutes. Stir and cook a couple more minutes until the onion is soft and opaque.

If adding optional vegetables, chop up to 2 cups [200g] of vegetables into small pieces and put them in now, cooking with lid on for 4 minutes, stirring occasionally. Lower heat slightly if it starts cooking too quickly (i.e. browning). Stir in crushed tomatoes and cook for another 5 minutes, stirring frequently.

Meanwhile, combine tomato paste, stevia and vegetable stock in a medium bowl. Add to the stovetop mixture and cook slowly for another 8 minutes. At this point, you can lower the heat to simmer and let the flavours develop for approximately 20 minutes, if you prefer. Either way, taste before serving to check the balance of flavours—you may need to add more stock or more stevia to your liking.

Just before serving, remove from heat and stir in basil leaves. Ladle soup into bowls and if using shredded cheese, top soup in each bowl with 1 tablespoon cheese.

Creamy Cauliflower Soup with Parmesan Crisps   (Serves 6)

1 head of cauliflower (medium size)
2 tablespoons extra virgin olive oil
1 small onion, chopped
2 cloves garlic, minced (2 teaspoons)
4 cups [1 litre] chicken stock, homemade (p. 169) **or** good quality brand such as Imagine (i.e. natural ingredients, no MSG, no refined sugar)
½ cup [50g] Parmesan cheese, finely grated
sea salt **and** pepper to taste
½ tsp nutmeg
⅓ cup [80ml] cream, preferably organic
Optional garnish: ½ cup [80g] green onions, chopped

Parmesan Crisps

1 chunk of fresh Parmesan cheese, about 8 ounces [100g]

Cut cauliflower right down the center for easy removal of the leaves and thick core. Coarsely chop flowerettes, and set aside. Heat the olive oil in a large saucepan over medium heat; add the onion and garlic and cook until softened but not browned, about 4 minutes. Add the cauliflower and stock and bring to a boil. Reduce the heat to a simmer, cover, and cook until the cauliflower is very soft and falling apart, about 15 minutes. Remove from heat and, using a hand held immersion blender, puree the soup, or puree in small batches in a blender and return it to the pot (see **NOTE**). Add the Parmesan, nutmeg and cream stirring until smooth. Season to taste, with salt and pepper. Garnish each bowl with a couple of Parmesan Crisp shards and a tablespoon of green onion.

To make **Parmesan Crisps**, preheat the oven to 350°F [180°C]. Using a large-holed grater, coarsely grate Parmesan. Line a baking sheet with lightly oiled parchment paper. Spread the shredded cheese over the parchment paper in an even thin layer. Bake about 10 minutes until golden brown and crisp. Remove from oven and let cool 5 minutes. Break sheet of crisp cheese into large pieces.

NOTE: When blending hot liquids, remove liquid from the heat and cool for at least 5 minutes. Transfer liquid to a blender or food processor and fill no more than halfway. If using a blender, release one corner of the lid. This prevents the vacuum effect that creates heat explosions. Place a towel over the top of the machine, pulse a few times then process on high speed until smooth.

Vegetables

Greek Vegetable Medley   (Serves 2)

2 cups [200g] cauliflower, in flowerettes
2 cups [200g] zucchini [courgette], in 1 inch [2 cm] pieces
1 cup [100g] broccoli, in flowerettes
2 tablespoons olive oil
1 tablespoon lemon juice
1 teaspoon dried marjoram

In vegetable steamer basket, steam cauliflower for four minutes. Add zucchini and broccoli to basket and steam for an additional four minutes. While vegetables cook, whisk together oil, lemon juice and marjoram to make vinaigrette. When vegetables are done, lightly toss with vinaigrette and serve immediately.

Swiss Chard with Lemon   (Serves 3)

½ cup [65g] raw sunflower seeds
½ medium onion, chopped
1 tablespoon coconut oil
3 cups [90g] Swiss chard **or** other greens, chopped and still damp from washing
1 teaspoon lemon juice

In 350°F [180°C] oven, toast sunflower seeds for several minutes until golden brown. Set aside. In large frying pan, heat coconut oil and then sauté onion until soft. Add Swiss chard and salt and cook over medium heat until chard is limp (3-4 minutes). Remove from heat. Toss chard/onion mixture with sunflower and lemon juice. Serve immediately.

Corn with Lime and Onion (B)   (Serves 2)

3 cups [485g] corn, frozen **or** fresh
1 small red onion, diced
juice of one lime (2 tablespoons)
1 tablespoon each cilantro **and** chervil, chopped

Steam corn and onion until tender crisp. Toss vegetables with remaining ingredients and serve immediately.

Spicy Popping Szechuan Beans

(Serves 4)

These beans were discovered at a restaurant, and the recipe recreated at home. At the restaurant it was served as an appetizer and eaten with chopsticks; sometime for fun, why not try that at home.

4 cups [400g] whole green beans, ends trimmed
2 tablespoons extra virgin olive oil
1 tablespoon shallots
1 clove garlic, minced (1 teaspoon)
2 tablespoons good quality Szechuan sauce (i.e. natural ingredients, low sugar content)
¼ teaspoon pepper
Optional: ½ teaspoon Serrano pepper, chopped width-wise into small circles

Steam green beans to just before they reach desired level of doneness (i.e. bright green, softened but still tender crisp). While beans are steaming, heat oil in frying pan on medium heat. Add shallots, garlic and peppers. Cook gently until softened. Add steamed beans to pan, topping with Szechuan sauce, and if extra spiciness is desired, the Serrano pepper rings. Stir to combine and cook for two more minutes to combine flavours, and until desired firmness of beans is reached. Remove to serving dish and top with pepper.

Easy Oven Roasted Vegetables

(Serves 4)

A flavourful and easy way to serve a variety of vegetables!

2 cups [200g] broccoli, in flowerettes
1 red onion, chopped in large pieces (i.e. in eights, then halved)
1 cup [100g] mushrooms, halved
1 cup [100g] zucchini [courgette], chopped in large pieces
1 red pepper, chopped in large pieces (i.e. in eights, then halved)
1 yellow pepper, chopped in large pieces (i.e. in eights, then halved)
¼ cup [60ml] extra virgin olive oil
handful basil leaves
sea salt **and** pepper to taste
½ teaspoon cumin

Preheat oven to 350°F [180°C]. Combine vegetables in a large roasting pan. Pour olive oil across vegetables and stir to coat. Stir in salt, pepper and cumin. Cover and cook for 17 to 20 minutes only so texture stays firm. Remove from oven. Stir in basil leaves and serve.

NOTE: For a wonderfully different flavour experience, substitute 2 tablespoons of balsamic vinegar or **BALSAMIC REDUCTION** (p. 160) for the cumin.

Stir-fried Broccoli with Garlic (Serves 4)

3 cups [300g] broccoli
3 cloves of garlic, thinly sliced width-wise
3 tablespoons extra virgin olive oil
sea salt **and** pepper to taste
¼ teaspoon hot pepper flakes

Trim broccoli into bite-sized pieces; include stem pieces as well, if desired. Heat oil in skillet over medium heat. Add garlic and hot pepper flakes, sauté for about 2 minutes, until garlic begins to brown. Add broccoli and cook with lid on, stirring occasionally. Serve while tender crisp.

Baked Tomatoes (Serves 2)

2 whole tomatoes
2 teaspoons pesto sauce, homemade **or** good quality store bought (i.e. natural ingredients, low sugar content)
4 teaspoons Parmesan cheese, grated

Place oven rack 4-6 inches [10-15 cm] from broiler. Preheat oven to 450°F. Cut tomatoes in half and lay cut-side up. Spread each tomato half with ½ teaspoon of pesto sauce. Top each tomato half with 1 teaspoon Parmesan cheese. Place tomatoes in a shallow baking dish or on an oven-roasting tray and cook for 6–8 minutes. If not browned on top at 6 minutes bake time, increase oven heat to broil for last minute or two.

Mashed Cauliflower (Serves 4)

An amazing substitute for mashed potatoes!

1 large head of cauliflower, in flowerettes
up to ½ cup [125ml] milk, preferably organic, as required
2 tablespoons each butter **and** sour cream **or** plain yogurt, preferably organic
sea salt to taste
pepper to taste
garlic powder to taste

Steam cauliflower until softened. Working in batches, blend cauliflower in a blender, adding milk as required, until it reaches a consistency similar to mashed potatoes. Once blended, remove to a large bowl and stir in butter, sour cream, salt and pepper and garlic powder.

Jicama-Pepper Salsa

(Makes 3 cups/250g)

A crunchy, exciting addition to Mexican or Asian inspired dishes.

2 cups [200g] jicama, peeled and diced
1 red pepper, diced
juice of one lime (2 tablespoons)
3 tablespoons cilantro, chopped
1 hot pepper (i.e. Thai, Serrano, Jalapeno), seeded and minced (use rubber gloves when mincing and avoid touching eyes)
sea salt **and** pepper to taste

Combine ingredients in a medium sized bowl and serve as a condiment for dishes such as **TACO SALAD**, **SOPA DE TORTILLA** or **ASIAN CHICKEN DRUMSTICKS**.

Fruits and Desserts

Pears in Raspberry Puree (B)   (Serves 2)

½ cup [75g] raspberries, fresh **or** frozen
½ cup [75g] black currants **or** blackberries, fresh **or** frozen
2 pears, halved and cored

If frozen, let berries thaw. Process berries in blender or puree with hand blender until smooth. Place two pear halves on each of two plates.

Drizzle berry sauce on pears and serve.

Fruit Soup (B)   (Serves 4)

2 cups [300g] pineapple, in chunks
2 cups [400g] cantaloupe, in chunks
1 pink grapefruit, sectioned
1 apple, cored and seeded
1 cup [100g] purple seedless grapes, whole
1 cup [150g] strawberries, quartered
Optional garnish: several whole strawberries and coconut strips

Process pineapple, cantaloupe and grapefruit in blender or food processor until smooth.

Pour blended fruit into a bowl and add apple, grapes and quartered strawberries. Garnish soup with whole berries and coconut and serve.

Icy Fruit Shake (B)   (Serves 2)

2 medium bananas, frozen in chunks
2 cups [500ml] almond **or** coconut milk
1 cup [150g] frozen berries **or** pineapple

Pulse bananas and berries or pineapple in food processor for 30 seconds. With processor on, add milk and blend until smooth. Add additional milk if mixture is too thick.

Serve immediately.

Yogurt/Kefir Smoothie (B)   (Serves 2)

2 cups [500ml] whole milk yogurt **or** kefir, preferably organic
2 tablespoons coconut oil
1 peach, frozen in chunks, about ¾ cup [100g]
¼ pineapple, in chunks, about 1 cup [150g]
Optional: ½ tablespoon good quality powdered greens supplement (i.e. no added chemicals or refined sugar)

Process ingredients in blender until smooth. For a thinner consistency, add a small amount of water.

Serve immediately.

Fruity Protein Shake (B)   (Serves 2)

3 tablespoons raw almonds
3 tablespoons raw sunflower seeds
3 cups [750ml] filtered water
1 fresh **or** frozen banana, in chunks
½ cup [75g] fresh **or** frozen blueberries
½ cup [75g] fresh **or** frozen raspberries
½ cup [75g] frozen cranberries

Process nuts and seeds in blender until coarsely ground. Slowly add water, then fruit and blend until frothy.

Serve immediately.

Berry Coconut Milk Shake (B)   (Serves 2)

5-6 ice cubes
2 cups [500ml] full fat coconut milk
1 cup [150g] fresh **or** frozen blueberries **or** raspberries

Process ice cubes in blender until coarsely chopped. Slowly add coconut milk and fruit; blend until mixed.

Serve immediately.

Maple Ricotta Pudding (Serves 1)

A quick and wonderful protein-based snack or dessert!

½ cup [125g] ricotta cheese, preferably organic
¼ teaspoon maple extract flavouring
up to ¼ teaspoon of stevia powder

Combine ricotta cheese and maple extract. Add stevia in tiny amounts to sweeten to desired taste.

This dessert is quite dense and filling and the recipe may be too large for a single serving. Either share the pudding or reduce ricotta cheese to ⅓ cup and add the other ingredients to taste.

Have some fun trying other flavours with this pudding (i.e. almond flavouring and slivered almonds, vanilla flavouring and a few shakes of unsweetened cocoa powder). On a night when it is a Sometimes Foods occasion, top with 4 or 5 small chocolate chips. Enjoy!

Chilled Espresso Custard (Serves 4)

1½ cups [375ml] 2% milk, preferably organic
2 eggs, preferably free range, beaten
stevia powder to sweeten
2 teaspoons espresso powder **or** instant decaf coffee
1 teaspoon vanilla extract
Optional garnish: cinnamon

In a medium bowl, whisk together all ingredients (except cinnamon) until well blended.

Divide mixture evenly between four 6-ounce [180ml] ramekins (custard cups) and place in a 10 inch [22 cm] stovetop skillet.

Pour water into skillet and around the ramekins, up to ½ inch [1 cm] from the tops of the ramekins. Bring water to boil over high heat. Once water is boiling, reduce heat to low, cover and simmer for 10 minutes.

Remove the cups from the skillet, cool and cover with plastic wrap. Refrigerate for 3 hours or until chilled through.

Garnish with a sprinkle of cinnamon.

Appendix 1

KIB Body Type Survey

Directions:

- ❑ Complete the following survey with your child, circling only one answer per question.
- ❑ Realize there are no right or wrong answers, only different answers based on the body type of your child.
- ❑ Ask your child's opinion as to the most accurate answer, but, as well, temper the answer with your own observations.
- ❑ Take time to thoroughly read the questions and, because some of them may deal with topics you have not previously thought about, carefully consider the answers. Conversely, however, do not ponder the questions too long; usually the first "gut response" is the most accurate.
- ❑ If you are unable to answer some questions because your child has not had the experience the question asks about (i.e. a vegetarian meal, eggs for breakfast), then leave the question, give the experience a try (i.e. a bean chili), see how your child feels and then answer the question.
- ❑ Because some characteristics apply only to a couple of body types, several of the questions have only two answer choices. Circle the one that more closely describes your child.
- ❑ The more survey questions that are answered, the more accurate indication you will have of body type. However, if none of the answers to a question even come close to describing your child, leave that question unanswered.
- ❑ When the survey is complete, follow the instructions at the end to determine body type.
- ❑ The questions are phrased as being read by your child. If you are reading them to your child, please re-frame the questions accordingly.

Appetite

1) My hunger feelings tend to be:

    A) Weak and/or don't get hungry very often.
    B) Strong and/or happen a lot and can feel out of control.
    C) Medium strength and/or not at all out of control.

2) When it comes to food:

    A) I hardly ever think about it and some times might even forget to eat.
    B) I think about it a lot; I really love and enjoy food and it is a big part of my life.
    C) I think about it sometimes and like food, but it is not a huge part of my life.

3) At meal or snack time:

A) I usually do not eat that much, probably less than most people I know.
B) I usually eat a lot (or would like to eat a lot if I was allowed).
C) I usually eat an average amount of food, about the same as most people I know.

4) To feel full:

A) I do not need to eat much.
B) I need to eat a lot.
C) I need to eat an average amount.

5) If I could choose how often I ate:

A) I would like 2-3 meals/day and maybe a little snack or two.
B) I would like to eat often throughout the day with three big meals and large snacks.
C) I would like 3 medium sized meals and maybe a snack or two.

6) If I eat a meal with no meat (i.e. vegetarian) such as a bean chili or big salad with nuts:

A) I feel full enough and do fine until my next meal or snack.
B) I feel there is something missing in my meal and/or feel hungry soon after eating.
C) I feel o.k. after a meal with no meat, but I like having meals with meat sometimes too.

7) If I miss a meal:

A) I do OK and find missing a meal does not really bother me.
B) I do not do well and can feel cranky, weak and/or tired.
C) I do fairly well but do not really feel as well as if I'd had a meal.

Food Preferences

8) If I have cravings, they are more often for:

A) Light foods such as vegetables, fruits or crackers.
B) Heavy or fatty (greasy) foods such as peanuts, beef jerky, cheese and potato chips.
C) I do not really have cravings for any type of food.

9) When it comes to salt:

   A) I almost never put salt on my food or only put a tiny bit of salt on my food.
   B) I often add salt to my food and can crave salty foods.
   C) I sometimes add salt to my food.

10) When it comes to potatoes:

   A) I do not really care for them all that much.
   B) I love them and would eat them often if I could.
   C) I do not really have a preference; I like them fine but am fine without them too.

11) When it comes to fatty (greasy) foods:

   A) I do not enjoy or even really like fatty foods.
   B) I really love and/or crave the taste and feel of fatty foods (i.e. cheese, potato chips, rich meat dishes or creamy sauces).
   C) I prefer foods that are not too fatty or don't mind having fatty foods once in awhile.

12) My favourite types of snacks are:

   A) Sweet or light snacks such as fresh fruit, trail mix (nuts and dried fruit) or veggies and dip.
   B) Heavier snacks that aren't sweet, such as potato chips or nachos or wings.
   C) I do not really have a favourite. I like sweet snacks and salty snacks too.

13) If I could choose whichever piece of a roast chicken I wanted:

   A) I would choose a lighter piece like the breast.
   B) I would choose a darker piece like a thigh or drumstick.
   C) I could eat either type of chicken meat and enjoy it.

14) My favourite breakfast foods that I feel best on are:

   A) Lighter foods such as granola, toast and fruit or a fruit/yogurt smoothie.
   B) Heavier foods such as eggs, sausages and/or bacon.
   C) Medium foods such as cereal and milk or toast and peanut butter.

15) If I go to a buffet and can choose any food I like, I would likely choose:

   A) No meat or lighter meat like chicken breast, salad, rice and vegetables and a fruit tart.
   B) Lots of different kinds of meats, a few cooked vegetables, potatoes and gravy and maybe cheesecake.
   C) Almost equal parts meats, raw and cooked vegetables and pastas or rice and then maybe a dessert.

16) If I am offered a sweet dessert like cake, cookies or candies:

A) I usually say, "Yes," as I really like desserts and feel the meal is not quite complete without a sweet treat at the end.
B) I usually say, "No," as I would rather have another helping of meat or potatoes and gravy or a salty snack later on.
C) I sometimes say, "Yes" and sometimes say "No."

17) If I choose a dessert, I usually choose:

A) Lighter desserts such as cookies, fruit pies and cakes.
B) Heavier, fatty types of desserts like cheesecake or cream-filled pastries.

Energy

18) My energy is usually:

A) Higher than most people.
B) Lower than most people.
C) About the same as most people.

19) If I eat a fatty meal like ribs and vegetables with cream sauce:

A) It makes me feel tired and/or feeling too full.
B) It makes me feel happy and energized.
C) It usually doesn't change my energy levels much one way or the other.

20) If I eat a vegetarian meal of pasta with tomato sauce or a veggie wrap:

A) I feel good in my energy and mood.
B) I feel hungry soon after eating and I can also get tired, moody and cranky.
C) I usually do not feel much of a change in mood or energy.

21) When it comes to red meats like roast beef, meatballs, bacon, lamb or pork chops:

A) I do not really like them. They make me tired or moody.
B) I really like them and find they give me energy and make me feel good.
C) I enjoy small amounts of meat but do fine without it too.

22) If I eat a sweet such as candy, a cookie or a piece of cake all by itself:

A) I do o.k. and generally do not notice much shift in mood or energy.
B) I do not do very well, my energy can drop, I might get cranky and might have cravings for another sweet.

Emotions

23) My family and best friends would say that I show my emotions:

A) Rarely and carefully (i.e. don't usually let many people know how I am feeling).
B) Easily and openly (i.e. pretty much everyone around me would know how I was feeling).
C) Fairly easily (i.e. some people would know how I was feeling).

24) My family and best friends would say I am:

A) Shy, quiet and a bit of a loner.
B) Friendly, talkative or maybe even loud.
C) Pretty friendly but like my quiet times too.

25) If I am at a party:

A) I can feel a bit awkward or that I don't fit in, and may leave early.
B) I am often the "life of the party" and love to talk and hang out with friends.
C) I am neither a bit awkward nor the "life of the party" but somewhere in between.

26) If I eat something and it changes my mood:

A) My moods get better after eating foods like fruits, vegetables and whole grains, and, maybe not right away, but within maybe an hour, get worse after eating things like red meat and heavier, greasy foods.
B) My moods get better after eating foods like meat, cheese, or nuts and, maybe not right away, but within maybe an hour, get worse after eating things like pasta, bread and fruits.
C) Food doesn't seem to change my moods.

27) I like it best when my life is:

A) Planned and orderly, and I know what I'm doing next.
B) Unplanned and flexible, where anything could happen next.
C) Planning is fine, but I like a little flexibility and doing something spur of the moment as well.

Physical Characteristics

28) My extra weight is:

A) I usually don't have extra weight.
B) Pretty well everywhere on my body, but more of it seems to be in my stomach area.
C) Pretty evenly spread around my body.

29) Lots of people in my family are:

A) More thin than most people.
B) More overweight than most people and might even be really overweight.
C) About average weight.

30) My eyes are often:

A) Dry.
B) Moist and get teary sometimes (when I'm not crying).

31) My fingernails are usually:

A) Thick, strong and hard.
B) Thin and easily split or bend.

32) No matter what color my skin is, it is usually:

A) Pale or washed out looking.
B) Reddish or flushed.
C) Neither pale nor flushed.

33) My skin is usually more:

A) Dry and/or chapped.
B) Moist.
C) Balanced (i.e. neither dry/chapped or moist).

34) If I get an insect bite:

A) My reactions (i.e. bite mark or pain or swelling) are mild and usually go away quickly.
B) My reactions (i.e. bite mark or pain or swelling) are quite strong or long lasting.
C) My reactions (i.e. bite mark or pain or swelling) are average in how strong they are and how long they last.

35) My bowel movements:

    A) Are not very regular and I might go a day or two without having a movement.

    B) Happen regularly and are often 3 or more times/day.

    C) Happen regularly and 1-3 times/day.

36) When it comes to allergies:

    A) I have no allergies that I know of.

    B) I have allergies (especially seasonal ones like hay fever).

Sleep Patterns

37) I sleep better if my bedtime snack is:

    A) A lighter food higher in grains or fruit (i.e. an apple or a couple of whole grain crackers).

    B) A heavier food, higher in protein and fat (i.e. a chunk of cheese or a handful of nuts).

    C) Kind of bedtime snack does not make a difference in how I sleep.

38) I sleep better after a dinner of:

    A) More starchy, carbohydrate-rich foods than protein-rich foods (i.e. chicken Caesar with a little chicken and lots of vegetables and croutons).

    B) More protein-rich foods than carbohydrate-rich foods (i.e. a steak, salad and a little rice).

    C) The kind of dinner does not make a difference in how I sleep.

39) Sweet bedtime snacks (cookies, candy, fruit sticks, glass of juice):

    A) I do fine on a sweet bedtime snack.

    B) A sweet bedtime snack can make it hard for me to fall asleep or stay asleep.

40) If I have insomnia (a hard time falling asleep or staying asleep):

    A) It is never really caused by hunger or needing to eat something.

    B) It can be caused by hunger or needing to eat something.

Miscellaneous

41) If I had my choice of climate (i.e. weather, temperature) to live in I would prefer:

A) A warmer or hot climate as I often feel cold and/or do not really like the cold.
B) A cooler climate as I do not really like heat.
C) Either is OK as I do fine no matter what the temperature.

42) When it comes to exercise:

A) I really like it; I am happy to exercise and miss it when I don't exercise.
B) I really do not much like it; it feels almost like a chore.
C) I like exercise but do not mind when I miss it.

43) If I have to exercise:

A) I do not mind team sports, but I also really like exercising on my own.
B) I would rather exercise in a group (i.e. biking with friends or taking a swimming class or team sports) where I can hang out with and talk with friends.
C) It does not make a difference to me whether I exercise by myself or in a group.

44) Before or after exercise, I feel better if I:

A) Eat or drink a starchy snack such as a fruit or fruit juice or crackers.
B) Eat or drink a protein-rich snack such as a yogurt smoothie or nuts.
C) Eat or drink a snack that contains both carbohydrate-rich foods (i.e. fruit) and protein-rich foods (i.e. nuts).

45) If I were to gain more weight it would likely be:

A) By eating too many fats and heavier protein-rich foods such as cheese and meats
B) By eating too many starchy foods such as fruits, fruit juices, breads, pasta and other grains.

Total your child's A) answers, B) answers and C) answers. If your child scored the highest number of answers in the A) category, he or she is a Carbohydrate Body Type. If your child scored the highest number of answers in the B) category, he or she is a Protein Body Type. If your child scored the highest number of answers in the C) category, he or she is a Mixed Body Type.

If your child scored more than 22 points in the A) category he or she is an Extreme Carbohydrate Type and if your child scored more than 22 points in the B) category he or she is an Extreme Protein Type. While *KIB*'s body typing information is pertinent to all children in the program, it is particularly important that Extreme body types closely follow recommended *Fuel Mix Guidelines*.

Appendix 2

Fuel Mix Guidelines

The basic body typing information in the **B**-Body Type chapter (p. 23) is enough to get families started on **Find Your BALANCE**. However, as you and your child begin the transition to **Build Your BALANCE** it is helpful to look at additional material that will help your child determine a more exact ratio of the essential macronutrients—protein-rich foods, carbohydrate-rich foods and healthy fats—that are the best fuel mix for his particular body type. These food component ratios are how he will make up his mealtime plate and will determine his optimum snack foods.

Carbohydrate Body Types will have concentrated on the vegetable sources of protein-rich foods (i.e. seeds, legumes, nuts) and lighter white meats and fish in **Find Your BALANCE**, and in **Build Your BALANCE** will be ready to add in the food groups they need to eat in a higher percentage—starchy vegetables, grains and fruit. A good starting place ratio-wise is 25% protein-rich foods, 40% vegetables, 5% fats and 30% high fibre starchy vegetables, grains and fruit.

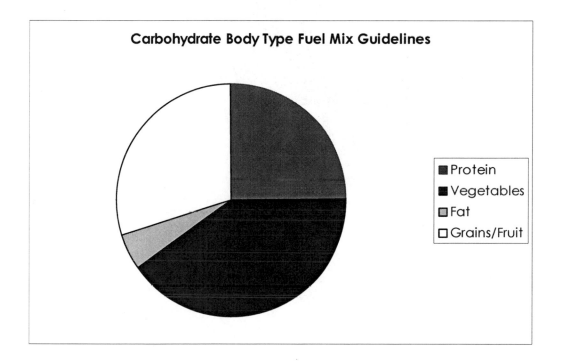

Mixed Body Types generally find that an approximately 50/50 ratio of protein-rich foods and fats/starchy vegetables, grains, vegetables and fruit keeps them at optimal weight and health. Therefore, once they have completed **Find Your BALANCE** that means approximately 40-50% of their meal will consist of protein-rich foods and fats, with the other 50-60% of the meal consisting of low starch vegetables, starchy vegetables, grains and possibly a fruit.

A good starting place ratio-wise is 40% protein-rich foods, 34% vegetables, 7% fats and 19% high fibre starchy vegetables, grains and fruit.

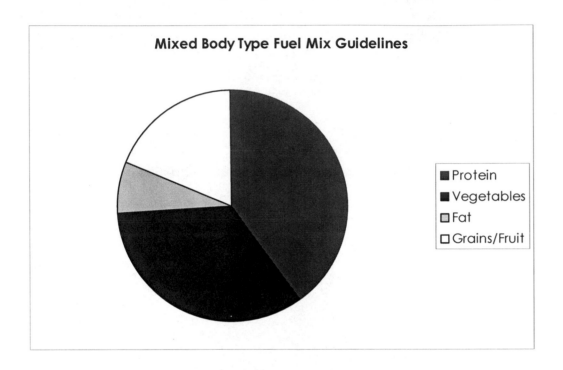

Protein Body Types will have found **Find Your BALANCE** foods in general produced a good response in their bodies; now the key is to slowly add in their cautionary food groups—starchy vegetables, grains and fruit—and, even in **Keep Your BALANCE**, to have them as only a small percentage (i.e. 10-20%) of each meal. A good starting place ratio-wise is 45% protein-rich foods, 30% vegetables, 10% fats and 15% starchy vegetables, high fibre grains and fruit.

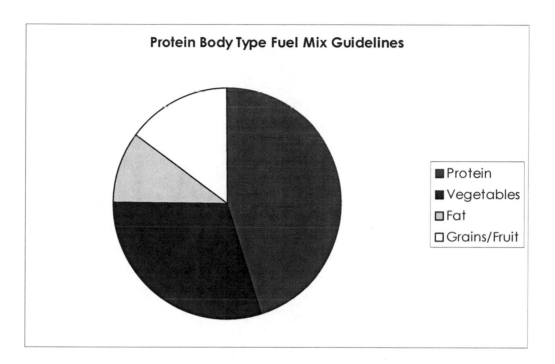

With all body types, it is important to add in cautionary foods in a manner that supports any additional weight loss or health gains needed. In **Keep Your BALANCE**, cautionary and Some-times Foods are eaten in amounts that allow a body to maintain appropriate weight and health. As the previously mentioned nursery rhyme, "Jack Sprat could eat no fat, his wife could eat no lean, and so betwixt the two of them, they licked the platter clean," so aptly describes, every body is different.

As hopefully Jack and his wife did, however, your child will need to monitor his body symp-toms after eating. The *Fuel Mix Guidelines* are just that—**guidelines**. The following Body Clues will ensure you know how to monitor symptoms such as mental clarity, moods and energy, and can then adjust your child's fuel mix to contribute to his reaching optimum health.

Fine-tuning the *Fuel Mix Guidelines*

For the first few weeks of **Build Your BALANCE**, one to two hours after each time your child eats, do a quick check with him through the following *Fuel Mix Evaluation Chart*. If you check all Right Fuel Mix body responses, continue with the proportions of each food group you are using. If you check any Wrong Fuel Mix responses, refer to the previous Body Type *Fuel Mix Guidelines* charts and make adjustments to the type of food groups or the proportion of food groups being eaten.

Fuel Mix Evaluation Chart

Body Clues	Right Fuel Mix	Wrong Fuel Mix
Physical—Energy	-Feel a sense of restored energy after eating -The energy is stable, consistent and lasting -Feel an overall sense of physical well-being	-Feel no increase in energy after eating -Feel an increased sense of lethargy or exhaustion -Feel increased drowsiness or sleepiness -Feel an energy increase, but it is a jittery, frantic and/or wired type of energy -Feel increased energy, but it overlays a sense of exhaustion
Physical—Hunger	-Feel comfortably full and satisfied -Feel free of sugar/refined grain cravings -Feel free of hunger for the next 2-4 hours	-Feel hungry although physically there may be a sense of fullness -Do not feel satisfied -Feel a need for a sweet end to the meal -Feel hungry soon after the meal
Physical—Bloating	-Feel no sense of bloating, gas, uncomfortableness in stomach region	-Feel bloated and/or gaseous and/or a sense of uncomfortableness in stomach region
Emotional—Mood	-Feel emotionally balanced -Feel positive -Feel calm, patient	-Feel emotionally imbalanced or out of sorts -Feel low, blue or somewhat negative -Feel irritated or impatient
Mental—Clarity	-Feel mentally clear and can easily concentrate -Feel mentally sharp	-Feel mentally scattered or without easy focus -Feel mentally slow

Appendix 3

Label Reading Clues

Understanding how to read food labels—both the general nutritional claims information written on food packaging as well the actual ingredient list and Nutritional Facts table—is an important skill that can positively impact family health. Food labels help us see if the types of ingredients we are trying to include more often in our diet are contained in plentiful supply in a food product. They also help us determine whether or not the product contains anything family members might be allergic to and alert us to ingredients we may want to minimize or avoid.

General Nutritional Claims

Provided they meet Health Canada regulations for criteria and wording, food manufacturers can make two types of general nutritional claims: nutrient content claims and health claims (similar guidelines exist in the U.S.). Nutrient claims (i.e. no sugar added, sodium free) are "micro" based in that they help us look at one ingredient in the food. You still need to look at the Nutrition Facts table to get specific information about the nutrient in the nutritional claim but because a claim has been made, you know that information about that particular nutrient will appear in the table. Common nutrient claims include:

- ❑ *Free*—A nutritionally insignificant amount as in "sodium free": less then 5 mg sodium per serving.
- ❑ *Low*—Associated with a very small amount of a nutrient as in "low fat": 3 g fat or less per serving.
- ❑ *Reduced*—At least 25% less of a nutrient compared with a similar product as in "reduced in calories": at least 25% less calories/energy than the food to which it is compared.
- ❑ *Source*—Associated with a significant amount as in "source of fibre": 2 g fibre or more per serving.
- ❑ *Light*—If referring to a nutrient, the term is allowed on foods that are either **reduced** in fat or **reduced** in calories/energy as in "light in calories." Light can also refer to a feature of the food such as light in color, but this must be explained on the label.

Health Claims

A health claim makes a link between a certain food or nutrient and a health condition, and must be supported scientifically. Regulations are constantly being evaluated and amended, but currently there are only a limited number of permitted claims describing the relationship between a food/nutrient and a health condition:

- ❑ A healthy diet low in sodium and high in potassium may reduce the risk of high blood pressure.
- ❑ A healthy diet adequate in calcium and vitamin D may reduce the risk of osteoporosis.
- ❑ A healthy diet low in saturated and trans fat may reduce the risk of heart disease.

❑ A healthy diet rich in a variety of vegetables and fruit may help reduce the risk of some types of cancer.

❑ Maximal fermentable carbohydrates in gum, hard candy or breath-freshening products may reduce the risk of dental caries.

Ingredient Lists

Any food product that has more than one ingredient must have an ingredient list that contains all the ingredients in that product. Foods are listed in order by weight, from most weight to least weight. In general, stay away from food products with lengthy ingredient lists. Often the list is long because it contains a variety of additives or sugars or artificial ingredients.

Ingredient	Alternate Ingredient Terms
Fat	Glycerides, glycerol, esters, vegetable shortening.
Saturated fat	Tallow or beef fat, lard, suet, chicken fat, bacon fat, butter, coconut or coconut oil, hydrogenated fats and oils, cocoa butter, palm or palm kernel oil, powdered whole milk solids.
Trans fat	Hydrogenated or partially hydrogenated fats and oils.
Sodium	Salt, monosodium glutamate, baking powder, baking soda, disodium phosphate, sodium bisulfate, brine, garlic salt, onion salt, celery salt, soy sauce, tamari, sodium alginate, sodium benzoate, sodium hydroxide, sodium propionate.
Sugar	Brown or white sugar, beet sugar, corn sugar, corn syrup, confectioner's sugar, powdered sugar, turbinado, high-fructose corn syrup and sugar cane syrup. Table sugar is sometimes listed by its chemical name—**sucrose**. Chemical names for other sugars include **lactose** (milk sugar) and **fructose** (fruit sugar). The "ose" ending is a hint that the ingredient is the chemical name for a type of sugar. Other "ose" sugars include **glucose** (also called **dextrose**), **levulose** and **maltose**. Sugar is also sometimes listed as Sucanat, Demerara, molasses, malt syrup, maple syrup, honey, barley syrup, rice syrup, unrefined cane sugar, cane juice, raw sugar and fruit juice concentrate. These sweeteners may be less refined (i.e. closer to original form, may have more nutrients) but they are still a form of sugar and should be eaten in moderation.
Sugar alcohols	Isomalt (palatinit), lactitol, mannitol, maltitol, sorbitol, xylitol (xylitol is an acceptable sugar).

As well, pay attention to the types of ingredients. If they have long, chemical-sounding names, they are often either something that is not a "real" food or something that is not very close to its original form. Just because a name is unfamiliar, however, does not mean it is unsafe—ascorbic acid for example is simply vitamin C—but if you do not know what it is or what it can potentially do in your body, check it out before you eat it.

Because manufacturers can list ingredients by a variety of names it is important to both recognize what the generic ingredient is and pay attention to the cumulative volume of the ingredient terms that can be used for common ingredients.

Where's the sugar?

Want to know how many teaspoons of sugar are in a particular food product? One teaspoon of granulated white sugar is approximately 4.2 grams. To figure out how many spoonfuls of sugar are in a soda containing 44 grams of sugar, you would divide 44 by 4.2. That is over 10 teaspoons of sugar— about the maximum daily recommended amount. Makes a glass of homemade lemonade with stevia look pretty good!

DIGGING DEEPER-HFCS (Corn Sugar) and Fructose

High fructose corn syrup (HFCS), labeled glucose/fructose in Canada and isoglucose or glucose-fructose syrup in Europe, is the number one source of calories in the US. HFCS is the name for corn syrups that have undergone processing to increase their fructose content and are then mixed with pure corn syrup to reach a final product. Some research indicates HFCS is metabolized like table sugar and honey, and can be safely consumed in moderation. Other studies, however, show that HFCS is not recognized by the body in the same way as other sweeteners (i.e. does not stimulate insulin secretion or increase leptin production or suppress production of ghrelin, does not trigger satiety, does not metabolize to blood glucose) but instead is converted to triglycerides or is stored as visceral fat.

Fructose, though often thought of as naturally sourced and less processed, is also of concern. When stripped of the vitamins, minerals, fibre and phytochemicals that are a natural part of fruit, fructose is left without the important nutrients that help balance its rapid metabolism. In the absence of those nutrients, fructose consumption can lead to insulin resistance, increased triglyceride levels and increased visceral fat.

Research seems to show then, that increased links between ill health and sugar intake over the past few decades in North America are not simply connected to an increase in amount of total sugar ingested. Instead, while increased sugar intake of any type is of concern, increased fructose and HFCS intake is of particular concern, and both fructose (other than in modest, body type appropriate amounts of fruit) and HFCS should be placed on your family's "never" or "almost never" list.

Where's the salt?

While everyone's need for sodium intake is slightly different, most sources recommend a daily intake of between 1600-2500 mg (2400 mg is the sodium content of about a teaspoon of table salt—sodium chloride). Be sure to include **all** salt and sodium consumed, including sodium used in cooking, in packaged or restaurant foods and at the table.

Where's the Monosodium Glutamate (MSG)?

Many people experience negative symptoms when ingesting MSG (salt of the amino acid, glutamic acid) or are trying to avoid this ingredient, which is often used as a flavour enhancer. Need help in figuring out if your food product contains MSG? Take a look at the following lists of definite and possible sources of MSG.

Definite Sources of MSG

autolyzed yeast	hydrolyzed protein
calcium caseinate	sodium caseinate
gelatin	yeast extract

Possible Sources of MSG

textured protein	stock
carrageenan	barley malt
vegetable gum	malt extract
seasonings	malt flavouring
spices	whey protein
flavourings	whey protein isolate
natural flavourings	whey protein concentrate
chicken flavouring	soy protein
beef flavouring	soy protein isolate
pork flavouring	soy protein concentrate
smoke flavouring	soy sauce
bouillon	soy extract
broth	

DIGGING DEEPER-MSG

While KIB's "eating real food" stance rules out MSG intake, it is not simply the desire to minimize altered concentrations of even naturally occurring compounds that has MSG on the avoid list.

Animal research conducted by Dr. John Olney in 1969 and confirmed in numerous studies since, showed that exposing babies prenatally or as newborns to MSG results in gross obesity.

According to experts such as Dr. Russell Blaylock (*Excitotoxins: The Taste That Kills*), the culprits seem to be excitotoxins—toxic chemicals that excite brain cells to death—like glutamate (found in MSG) and aspartate (found in Aspartame™). Foods containing MSG or highly processed milk and soy protein—processing breaks down those proteins, releasing high levels of glutamate and aspartate—can damage an unprotected part of the brain that is responsible for controlling hunger and satiety.

It seems particularly important to eliminate MSG intake prenatally and up to age three but two other facts discovered while researching MSG intake with animals show we should all stay clear:

1) Animals studied began to prefer sweeter, more carbohydrate-rich foods to healthier foods.

2) The MSG preferentially produced visceral (i.e. abdominal) fat.

Nutritional Facts Table

This table is found on most packaged food products and contains three types of information: serving size, number of calories per serving size and nutrient information of the same 13 nutrients. It is a great source of information for looking at the general nutritional quality of the product as it gives you the "macro" picture of what a product contains. Key factors to consider when reading Nutrition Facts tables are:

Nutrition Facts

Serving Size 1 ounce   Servings in bag 4

Amount Per Serving

Calories 155	Calories from Fat 93

	% Daily Value*
Total Fat 11g	16%
Saturated Fat 3g	15%
Trans Fat	
Cholesterol 0mg	0%
Sodium 148mg	6%
Total Carbohydrate 14g	5%
Dietary Fiber 1g	5%
Sugars 1g	
Protein 2g	

Vitamin A	0%	• Vitamin C	9%
Calcium	1%	• Iron	3%

* Percent Daily Values are based on a 2,000 calorie diet. Your daily values may be higher or lower depending on your calorie needs.

Serving size: When looking at the amount of calories or the % Daily Value of a nutrient, be sure to look at the serving size on which the information is based. The amount listed helps you make a good choice as to how much of a food to eat as well as helps in planning where you will get the mainstay of your foods from each day (i.e. many fruit and veggie bars contain 2 servings of produce, but they contain 29g of sugar; because it is a good idea to keep your daily intake of fructose to less than 15g, that means it is generally wiser to choose two servings of fresh vegetables and avoid the sugar hit).

Calories: These can be an important consideration when making daily food choices. While *KIB* focuses mainly on quality, type of food group, personalized Fuel Mix and proper food portions (i.e. eating for Comfortable Fullness) if, despite increased exercise, weight issues continue to be a challenge, it can also be important to more carefully look at the caloric value of the food types being chosen.

Nutrients: If you are eating to increase (i.e. calcium) or decrease (i.e. sodium) certain types of nutrients, careful reading of the Nutritional Facts table makes it easy to choose foods with a higher or lower % Daily Value of the nutrients you are trying to increase or decrease. As well, pay attention to the amount of trans fat in a product. That is one ingredient that should be on your family's "never" or "almost never" list.

DIGGING DEEPER
Label Reading

Some of the nutrition facts in this appendix were sourced at the Nutritional Labeling Information Centre. For additional helpful material, check out:
www.healthyeatingisinstore.ca (Canadian information) and
www.fda.gov/Food/LabelingNutrition/ConsumerInformation/UCM078889.htm (US information).

Appendix 4

KIB-Friendly Supplements

While *Kids in Balance* is predominantly and passionately a natural, whole foods-based program, I also recognize that with the physical, emotional and environmental stressors present today, dietary supplementation can be a wise choice. Research results and real life experience have shown that transitioning to a healthier weight and state is usually a more easily attainable goal if the right complement of nutrients is taken in—via diet and high quality supplements—on a daily basis. Therefore, while the *KIB* program can be undertaken and be highly successful with food supplying the sole source of nutritional intake, I recommend evaluating whether or not your child would benefit from intake of one or more of the following supplements. Take a look at the benefits provided by each supplement and determine whether you feel your child has any deficiencies in those areas. If so, add in correct amounts, per suggestions on product label, of the appropriate supplement. Alternatively, visit a holistic nutritionist or naturopathic doctor for personalized input.

Multi-Vitamin and Mineral Supplement—A good quality vitamin and mineral supplement or whole food product such as bee pollen or greens (supplements that contain a wide range of vitamins and minerals in a whole food base) is a helpful support for most children and adults. Sufficient intake of the wide range of vitamins and minerals our bodies require is essential for:

❑ Immune system functioning, energy and stamina.
❑ Sleep and sense of restfulness.
❑ Reduction in food cravings and healthy weight maintenance.

If you add a children's multi-vitamin or whole food product to your child's diet, source a good quality (i.e. avoid colouring, preservatives and refined sugars) chewable or encapsulated product through a natural supplement distributor or at a health food store.

Essential Fatty Acid Supplement—Many children and adults receive an inadequate dietary intake of the Essential Fatty Acids (EFAs) our bodies require to achieve optimal health. Because the body cannot make the "essential" nutrients it needs, those nutrients must be supplied through food or supplements. With current levels of ocean contamination, however, it is almost impossible to eat enough healthy fish to supply adequate amounts of EFAs. Therefore, along with a modest intake of fish (see www.oceansalive.org for good varieties and then eat 1-2 servings/week), include vegetarian forms of these nutrients (i.e. flax or walnuts) and consider supplementation. Among other key functions, EFAs help with:

❑ Mood stabilization, brain development and ability to learn.
❑ Pain and inflammation.
❑ Cardiovascular health.
❑ Immune system functioning.
❑ Health of hair and skin.
❑ Carbohydrate craving reduction.
❑ Cardiovascular health.
❑ Immune system functioning.

Two fatty acids—linoleic acid (LA), the "mother" omega-6 oil from which other omega-6 oils can be derived, and alpha linolenic acid (ALA), the "mother" omega-3 oil from which other omega-3 oils can be derived—are unable to be produced by the body and thus are deemed essential fatty acids (EFAs) that need to be supplied through diet. Because of many children's distaste for fish dishes, today's need to somewhat limit fish intake due to fish supply quality and the fact that not everyone does well on high amounts of vegetarian omega-3 food sources such as flax and walnuts, it is hard for a child's needs for omega-3 EFAs to be met through diet alone. Most children get an overly abundant amount of omega-6 oils such as canola, corn and soybean oil in their diet. However, as much of it comes in the form of trans or altered omega-6 fats there is often still a need to supplement with healthy, unadulterated versions of this EFA as well.

For additional information on EFAs check out Udo Erasmus' intensely detailed but excellent book, *Fats that Heal Fats that Kill* or *Know Your Fats: The Complete Primer for Understanding the Nutrition of Fats, Oils and Cholesterol* by Mary G. Enig.

❑ Hormone production, and insulin regulation and reduction. (Insulin is a hormone that thwarts the body's attempts to use fat for fuel and, in the presence of excess caloric intake/high blood sugar levels, can promote fat storage. High levels of insulin make it less likely the body will use stored fat as a fuel source. The balanced insulin levels that EFA supplementation promotes, allow for the release of stored fat and for more fat to be used for energy production.)

I recommend EFA supplementation with a liquid or capsule that has a linoleic acid (LA): alpha linolenic acid (ALA) ratio of between 1.5:1 and 2.5:1 in roughly the following amounts: 1 capsule per every 40 pounds of body weight or if in liquid form, 1 teaspoon per every 75 pounds of body weight. If you add EFAs to your child's regime, source a good quality LA/ALA product through a natural supplement distributor or at a health food store.

Probiotic Supplements—Probiotics is a general term for the families of helpful bacteria that inhabit the gut. One of the key roles of probiotics is to produce the enzymes that are responsible for digestion and assimilation of nutrients in the body. Without proper balance of healthful gut bacteria a body can begin to experience the myriad of health challenges that come along with nutritional deficiencies. Among other key health benefits, probiotics are important factors in maintaining healthy:

❑ Immune system functioning.
❑ Skin health.
❑ Hormone production and insulin regulation.
❑ Digestion, bowel functioning and bacteria balance in the gut.
❑ Food choices and body weight (i.e. reduces cravings and helps maintain proper appetite regulation).

If you add probiotics to your child's daily regime, first note that the many food products (i.e. yogurts, other dairy products) advertised as being high in probiotics do not generally contain a wide variety of strains of probiotic (i.e. often only lactobacillus acidophilus) nor enough probiotic to be a good supplemental source. Instead purchase a high quality probiotic (i.e. contains a high quantity of colony forming units [CFUs] and contains several strains of bacteria) through a natural supplement distributor or at a health food store.

Fibre—The indigestible parts of vegetables, legumes, nuts, seeds, grains and fruits play a large role in health maintenance. Following *KIB*'s recommended servings of vegetables, legumes, nuts and seeds in **Find Your BALANCE** and adding in small amounts of whole grains and fruits in **Build** and **Keep Your BALANCE** phases goes a long way to meeting daily fibre requirements. The right amount of fibre intake means more complete experience of fibre's many benefits:

- ❏ Supporting a smoothly functioning digestive system and keeping the bowels moving smoothly.
- ❏ Contributing to a sense of comfortable fullness and helping balance blood sugar levels.
- ❏ Playing a role in healthy cholesterol levels.
- ❏ Possibly giving protection against certain types of cancer.

Fibre can generally be divided into two types, soluble and insoluble, with many foods being rich in both types of fibre. Known mainly for its ability to help lower blood cholesterol levels, soluble fibre is found in higher concentrations in legumes, psyllium, apples, oats, nuts, barley, freshly ground flax seed or sesame seeds and citrus fruits. Soluble fibre includes the gum and pectin forms of fibre, and dissolves or softens in liquid to create a gel-like substance that can help with stool softening.

Insoluble fibre, found in the cellulose and lignin forms of fibre, has, as one of its main properties, the ability to retain water. More commonly used to help with constipation by speeding transit time, insoluble fibre is found naturally in a variety of foods including onions, greens, bananas, chicory root, celery, fruit skins, root vegetable skins, garlic and wheat (if your child has gluten or grain sensitivities, avoid adding increased amounts of foods such as wheat or oat bran).

Taking fibre in by whole foods seems to produce benefits beyond taking fibre components separately, therefore should there be times when additional fibre is needed in your child's diet, first start with upping his vegetable intake (per suggestions in the **Eat for Health** chapter p. 59) and ensuring refined grains and sugars have not crept back into your child's diet.

If it seems a supplemental form of fibre is needed, check out different varieties at your local health food store including those containing psyllium, inulin or PGX (Polyglycoplex®). With the latter, though PGX has been trialled on adolescents, until studies are done on younger children, if you choose to add PGX to your child's diet, I suggest keeping PGX usage to children 13 years of age and older. Regardless of type of fibre, add supplemental fibre slowly and with sufficient water intake to prevent gas, bloating, cramping or even increased constipation.

Amino Acid Supplements—Generally *KIB*'s dietary and lifestyle recommendations help balance blood sugar levels and contribute to mood stability in a way that minimizes or eliminates cravings. Occasionally, however, amino acid deficiencies will be of a depth that requires supplementation to settle cravings. For further information on amino acid deficiency symptoms see Julia Ross' *The Mood Cure* or *The Diet Cure*. If deficiencies are shown, work with an ND or nutritionist to determine type (i.e. 5-HTP) and dosage (i.e. usually ½ dose for children) of amino acid required.

Appendix 5

KIB on a Budget

Whether it is moving to a new home, changing jobs or schools, or getting ready for a shift of seasons, change can cost not only in time and energy expenditure but financially as well. While the *Kids in Balance* approach is simple, there will absolutely be some energy, time and dollar expenditure required when moving toward *KIB*'s lifestyle recommendations. With careful planning, however, it is possible to keep those changes within your family budget. Be wise, take the time to prepare well per the *Day-at-a-Glance Guidelines* and take heed of the following budget recommendations. Living well and eating well will cost. It should not, however, break the bank. And ultimately, your child's health and wellness results should prove the expenditures to have been very cost-effective choices!

The keys to successfully walking out the *KIB* approach, while effectively keeping within the family budget, are:

- ❑ Know what you have to spend.
- ❑ Substitute healthy choices for any current, costly unhealthy choices.
- ❑ Evaluate the best way for your family to incorporate each of the seven BALANCE solutions based on your budget.

Finally, recognize that virtually every weight loss program on the market is going to cost you money. Whether you are paying for packaged food, summer camps, supplements, gym membership or fees to attend weekly meetings, weight loss plans are generally not free. Finding one that is fully described in a helpful, low priced manual, that promotes the use of real food and that incorporates lifestyle change, rather than a quick fix mentality, however, is ultimately going to be the most cost effective way to have your child reach an appropriate weight in a healthy manner.

Many of the first six *KIB* solutions to childhood obesity, **B**-Body Type, **A**-Attitude, **L**-Laughter and play, **A**ctivity, a good **N**ight's sleep and **C**lean water cost almost nothing to implement. Determining your child's body type is as simple as completing the *KIB Body Type Survey* found on p. 179. **A**ttitude too is a freebie! While changing one's attitudes toward circumstances or getting a handle on the types of responses chosen in different situations can take effort, those attitudinal shifts cost nothing in terms of monetary expenditure.

The next four *KIB* solutions—**L**aughter and play, **A**ctivity, a good **N**ight's sleep and **C**lean water—are where families have a high degree of flexibility in the amount of money they choose to spend. If there is lots of room in the budget, families can spend spring break playing at Disneyland, set up a home gym with state-of-the-art equipment, buy EMF reducing devices to create an EMF–free zone in their house and get the latest, most effective water purification system on the market. Fortunately, none of those steps are necessary to have wonderful success with *Kids in Balance*.

The *KIB* approach works equally well even if your budget precludes the purchase of high-ticket items. Creating a climate of **L**aughter and play in your home takes nothing more than a family's willingness to learn some new card games, play a round of charades or borrow a few joke books and a funny video from the library. If your child is younger, filling up a "Tickle Trunk" with a selection of dress-up clothes and accessories from the local thrift shop is a great way to increase creativity and play.

Activity too, can be as simple as incorporating daily walks into the household routine. PACEing (p. 44) a couple of the walks each week and varying the route to avoid boredom costs nothing and goes a long way toward having your child achieve her goals. Your child can even do sets of stairs in your home (provided your home has more than one floor) or do a simple home exercise program (i.e. borrow the *Callanetics* book or videos by Callan Pinckney from the library for a great start). If your **Activity** budget has the room, add a little more variety by purchasing a good quality skipping rope or watching the classified ads for a used rebounder. You could even look at enrolling your child in a dance class or sports program. If those options seem outside your family's financial reach, be sure to check out community resources. Often there are subsidies or grants from local businesses to ensure all kids get an opportunity to be active.

Remember as well, to make some different choices with cash allocated elsewhere in the budget. If you regularly rent movies for family night, use that money to go on a family swim night; not only will you still get the benefit of family time, you will participate in some healthy physical activity and avoid the temptation of a poor choice of movie snack in the process.

While it is a great goal to have top quality room-darkening blinds and EMF-reducing devices on your child's cell phone or the family computer, even actions as simple as hanging a dark sheet over the window at night or removing electrical equipment (i.e. cell phones, digital alarms, radios, TVs) from your child's room help contribute to a good **Night's** sleep. And while getting to bed on time, like **Attitude**, costs in terms of effort and discipline, it too is a very inexpensive and effective support in your child's journey toward wellness.

Drinking sufficient tap water, one of the most cost effective beverages in most places in the world, is the place to begin with ensuring your child is well hydrated. Moving to even purer **clean** water, a simple container type filtration system (i.e. Brita™) is generally the least costly home water purification method. After that, the field is wide open both in type of purification system as well as in cost. If purchase of a more extensive water filtration system is something you are considering, look at:

- ❑ **Type of filtration system**—Investigate the pros and cons of various types of water filtration. For a head start in your research, note that based on my evaluation, I prefer the British Berkefeld portable gravity filtration, reverse osmosis, Santevia™ or MRET water purification systems to distillation or ionization.
- ❑ **Initial cost**—Systems vary widely in price, but remember sticker price is not everything. If you pay less for a system that has a shorter lifespan you may end up paying much more long term.
- ❑ **Replacement costs**—Most water systems have at least one or two parts that need regular maintenance (i.e. cleaning of the candles in a British Berkefeld system) or replacement of filtration cartridges. Be sure to factor in those time and money costs when determining which system is right for your family.

Because food is so vitally important and such a regular part of our day, *KIB*'s Eat for Health component has the potential to create the biggest shift in a family's budget, thus the amount of *KIB on a Budget* tips in this area. Fortunately, one of the many advantages of moving to a whole food dietary plan is that, in general, real unprocessed foods are less expensive than their processed and highly packaged counterparts. There are several types of natural foods that are more costly, however, and it is likely that good quality fats and dairy products will take a larger portion of your food budget than lesser quality products. And, if processed carbohydrate-based foods have been a large part of your grocery bill then adding in more quality protein-rich foods will have financial impact.

If you adopt the following suggestions, though, your family should be able to achieve increased health on a relatively similar dollar amount.

- ❑ Enjoy more slow food and less fast food. Eating dinner out almost always costs more than eating at home.
- ❑ Follow the same "slow food" principle at lunch, and brown bag it for both yourself and your child. Not only will the packed lunch cost less, in general, it will also be more nutritious and help keep you on the *KIB* program more easily.
- ❑ Watch your expenditures on snack breaks. Make your own iced rooibos or peppermint tea at home and transport it in a stainless steel container. Pair your beverage with homemade trail mix and you will have a great tasting snack-time-to-go at great savings.
- ❑ Buy in larger sizes, provided the unit price is better, and when possible, in bulk to avoid packaging. If budgetary restraint or pantry size means you do not have the ability to buy bulkier but smaller cost per volume sizes on your own, team up with a friend or neighbour. That way you expend the cost of a smaller size but reap the benefits of a better unit-priced larger purchase.
- ❑ To ensure that having more of an item in the house (i.e. a family pack of beef stew meat, larger wedge of Gouda cheese) does not lead to overeating or wastage, break the larger size package into appropriate meal-size quantities before storing separately or freezing, or prepare a double portion of a recipe and freeze half for later use.
- ❑ Check weekly grocery flyers for specials and check ingredients carefully; generic brands sometimes have the same or better ingredients and fewer additives than more expensive brands.
- ❑ Read labels to ensure you are getting both the best value for your food dollar and the best nutrition (see *Label Reading Clues*, p.191).
- ❑ Buy local. Food that is grown close to home keeps more of its nutritional value and costs less to transport than food shipped from afar. Buying food produced near you also supports the local economy.
- ❑ For the ultimate in eating local, grow your own vegetables and fruit. Even with limited garden space, certain vegetables (i.e. peppers, different varieties of lettuce, radishes), fruit (i.e. strawberries, tomatoes) and herbs (i.e. parsley, cilantro, chives, basil) can easily be grown in patio containers or a small raised bed.
- ❑ Find out when your favourite grocery store marks down its produce and baked goods, and make a note on your calendar to shop at that time. You will be able to spend less on an increased selection of slightly older but still healthy vegetables, fruits and sprouted whole grain breads.

- Likewise, check the yellow pages to see if you have a liquidation store nearby. Much of what these types of businesses stock comes from shops that have closed down, or retailers, manufacturers, wholesalers and distributors who have been left with cancelled orders, discontinued items, packaging glitches or changes, inventory overruns, or foodstuffs close to their best before date (watch dates!). Stock changes frequently and sometimes there may be nothing appropriate to your needs, but when liquidation stores have clearance sales on sprouted whole grain breads, healthy oils, natural turkey sausages or whole grain pasta, family taste buds and budget score big time. While freshest produce has the highest nutrient intake, even less crisp vegetables can still be used—think casseroles, stews or soup.
- Use coupons when applicable, but remember that most coupons are for overly processed or refined products that will not generally be on your grocery list.
- Healthy protein sources such as nuts, good quality cheese and meats are often the most expensive part of a food purchase, so remember that a little goes a long way. Protein-rich foods are very nutrient dense and when small amounts are paired with fibre-rich vegetables, nourishing fullness can be quite cost effective.
- Usually the least expensive way to buy poultry is to buy the whole bird. Roast the turkey or chicken for your first family meal, save the remaining meat to make a stir-fry or main dish salad and then prepare soup with the bones. Alternatively, cut smaller birds (i.e. chicken, duck) up yourself. That way you can freeze part of the meat for a meal at another time.
- Get a hold of some soup bones (i.e. buy them, or find a butcher store that gives them away) and make old-fashioned, long-simmering stock. See the *KIB* Recipe for stock on p. 169, or just "wing it." Making homemade stock can be as simple as putting bones, whole garlic cloves, a handful of parsley, a splash of apple cider vinegar and chunks of carrot, celery and onion in a stock pot, and covering with water up to 1 inch [2 cm] below the rim of the pot. Bring the water to a boil and then turn down to a simmer for 2-4 hours. Strain the liquid and voila, you have stock! The marrow in the bones provides great nutrients and according to Sally Fallon in *Nourishing Traditions* (where you can find a wide variety of stock recipes), the gelatin in meat stocks can help make even small amounts of protein be used more completely by the body. That means your homemade, stock-based soups can make cost effective amounts of protein-rich food go further in terms of healthful benefits!
- While animal-source protein foods such as meat, dairy products and eggs are usually more expensive than vegetable-source protein foods like chickpeas, lentils and sunflower seeds, remember that in order to reach optimal health, Protein Body Types need animal-source protein on a regular basis. In order to stretch food dollars, make ample use of protein-rich vegetable foods, but with a Protein Body Type child, be sure to top up vegetarian chilies, soups or stews with small amounts of ground beef, bison stew meat or strips of roast lamb. Your child will get the animal-source protein foods she needs for an optimum fuel mix but in an affordable way.
- As much as possible, avoid junk food! That way when your family makes the occasional Sometimes Foods choice you will be able to spend the money saved on junk food for small amounts of better quality Sometimes Foods such as a natural ice cream or fair-trade dark

chocolate. You will have appropriate amounts of Sometimes Foods that are a little better for you and still be able to stay on budget.

❑ While *KIB* families are encouraged to share the food planning, shopping and prepping load, be sure to distribute the grocery shopping task to family members who have had a nutrient dense and fibre-filled snack before entering the store. Hungry shoppers more easily get attracted to less-than-healthy food samples or attractive packaging and advertising for less-than-healthy food choices.

❑ And the #1 top *KIB* nutrition on a budget tip: menu plan, draw up a shopping list from the menu plan and stick to your shopping list! While occasionally sale priced items (i.e. chicken drumsticks) can be substituted for a regular priced item on your list (i.e. chicken thighs), usually straying for the grocery list means adding in "caught your eye" items that are less than healthy for either your body or your budget.

DIGGING DEEPER
Cooking 101

Not sure where to start with getting back to basics in the kitchen? Need some extra help in figuring out how to put tasty, healthy meals on the table at a reasonable cost? A good cookbook is a great place to begin.

Sandi Richard's *Cooking for the Rushed* series (www.cookingfortherushed.com/new/) is easily laid out, contains a minimum of processed foods (make appropriate substitutions if needed), and contains many recipes that are easily adapted for Protein and Balanced Body Types. The website also makes available, for a small fee, access to printable grocery lists.

Low-Glycemic Meals in Minutes (www.lowgimeals.com) by Laura Kalina & Cheryl Christian not only provides tasty and simple recipes but also teaches you how to prepare a week's worth of meals in two days/week. Protein Body Types will need to adjust dairy ingredients to moderate fat rather than the low fat recommended.

And when you are ready for more in-depth cooking preparation, wonderful nutritional information and a side dish of food "politics," be sure to check out Sally Fallon's cookbook based on the traditional food principles advocated by the Weston Price Foundation (www.westonaprice.org), *Nourishing Traditions, The Cookbook that Challenges Politically Correct Nutrition and the Diet Dictocrats*. After that title, need I say more!

Appendix 6

Family Activities

KIB kids generally fall between the ages of 5 and 18. They are amazing, unique individuals and all learn and grow in a variety of ways. Some do better reading along with mom or dad as parents go through the *Kids in Balance* program material. Others understand and respond better when the information is spoken aloud. Yet others need a more hands-on approach to learning about healthy living and need to be included on shopping trips and in food preparation.

Particularly with children 12 and under, a family game or activity that reinforces what is being spoken or read can be very helpful in moving the family along the wellness journey. The family activities that follow can be adapted to work with both children and teens, and don't be surprised if the grown-ups in a family learn something new as well!

Family Activity 1
Red Light, Green Light—Label Reading Activity

A fun way to learn how to read food labels.

What	How
Purpose	❑ Help family members grow in understanding of how to interpret food labels. ❑ Help family members make wise food choices based on the information on food labels.
Equipment	❑ Food labels, food packaging or even food items themselves from a variety of "great," "sometimes" and "almost never" food choices. ❑ Three sorting areas, one in each of the three traffic light colors—red, green and yellow (i.e. gift bags, boxes, placemats, baskets, pieces of construction paper). These will be used to hold labels/foodstuffs that "match" the types of food choices: green "great/have often" choices, yellow "sometimes" choices and red "almost never" choices. ❑ Review of *KIB's Label Reading Clues* (p. 191). ❑ Review of chapter 9 - Eat for Health (p. 59).
Directions	❑ Family members take turns choosing a label, food package or food item. ❑ A family member reads the label (or evaluates the food if it is a fruit or vegetable) and then decides if the food belongs in the red category as an "almost never" choice, in the yellow category as a "sometimes" choice or in the green category as a "great/have often" choice.
Tips	❑ While most families will have the same food stuffs and labels in the green category, different tastes, health challenges and cultural backgrounds may dictate variations in what items end up in the yellow or red categories (i.e. some families will have adults choosing wine as a "sometimes" item while others may have it as an "almost never" item; likewise interest in chocolate will vary from family to family). ❑ Remember that there will also be variations in body type between family members so certain family members may have whole grain products as a green item while others may have them as a yellow item.

Family Activity 2
Fuel Mix Fun—Body Type Activity

A helpful tool to determine the best fuel mix for each family member

What	How
Purpose	❑ Help family members grow in understanding of how and when to eat the right fuel mix for their body type and activity level. ❑ Help family members translate nutritional terms—protein, vegetables, fat, whole grains, fruit—into concrete examples of snacks and meals.
Equipment	❑ One plate for each family member. ❑ 10-12 paper circles, cut from heavy weight paper, to fit the plates. ❑ Magazines and grocery store flyers with large pictures of a wide variety of foods. You will need several pictures in each of the following categories: protein-rich foods, vegetables, fats, whole grains and fruits. ❑ Scissors or paper cutter and glue. ❑ Need a quick refresher on correct fuel mixes? Check out chapter 3 - Body Type and *Fuel Mix Guidelines*.
Directions	❑ Use heavy weight paper circles as a template to cut circles from the photos. Glue photos to the paper circles. ❑ Using scissors or a paper cutter, cut each food/paper circle into 6 equal pie-shaped sections and then categorize the sections into the *KIB* food groups—protein-rich foods, vegetables, fats, whole grains and fruit. ❑ Remind family members of the food fuel mix that works best for their body type and then have family members "build" meals from six of the pie-shaped sections that show good breakfast, lunch and dinner choices for their body type.
Tips	❑ Build a pre-sport or physical activity meal and a pre-sedentary evening meal. ❑ Look at both **Find Your BALANCE** and **Build Your BALANCE** options. ❑ Build a few "snack" plate alternatives. ❑ Can't remember all the options for the different food groups? Check out chapter 9 - **Eat for Health**, for help.

Family Activity 3
Family Meeting Time—Communication Activity

An effective plan to use when sorting through challenging situations

What	How
Purpose	❏ Help family members grow in their ability to discuss and role-play strategies for dealing with difficult situations. ❏ Help family members create a pressure point game plan as a method of keeping a child on the wellness journey despite circumstances and emotions.
Equipment	❏ All family members. ❏ A parent as facilitator/leader. ❏ A sense of calmness and humour.
Directions	❏ Outline the agenda item more specifically. ❏ Ask for input. ❏ Give your own input. ❏ Have family members express their goal(s) with regard to the agenda item (i.e. use proper goals/desires language, p. 33). ❏ List each member's goals on paper or a flip chart. ❏ Strategize ways to achieve the various objectives. ❏ Role-play any potential situations that may come up. ❏ Come to family agreement as to how the particular agenda item will be handled and affirm family members as to a job well done.
Tips	❏ Give advance warning as to when family meetings will take place. ❏ Let everyone have a chance to add to the agenda. ❏ Set the stage as to expectations on how family members present their points (i.e. one person speaks at a time, everyone stays on topic, family members—even if frustrated or angry—avoid derogatory or unkind remarks). ❏ Keep the tone positive (i.e. if need be, review Attitude information on re-framing, p. 41).

Family Communication Activity—An Example

As an illustration of how to more specifically conduct a healthy family meeting, take a look at the scenario on the following page. In this example the family is gathering together, a few weeks before the Christmas holidays, to discuss health goals in relation to the season, to identify potential challenges and to strategize solutions and game plans to navigate through those challenges.

As you work your way through the illustration, be aware that probably the most complex part of a family discussion is strategizing how to achieve various objectives, especially if the objectives are in conflict with each other.

For example, your child may want to attend one party where she does not have to worry too much about what she eats. Begin by defining what that means for your child. She may say that means she can eat whatever she wants and not think about her choices or their consequences. If one of her other objectives, however, is "I want to hold on to the success I have had so far in the *KIB* program," point out that these two objectives may be in conflict with each other.

Pose the question "If you could plan ahead on how to enjoy Sometimes Foods that night and minimize the negative effects, would that work for you?" If she agrees, discuss ways to make it possible for your child to relax a bit on food for one night and still hold on to her success. The solution the two of you come up with together could look like this:

- ❏ Have your child choose the social event, and plan to eat per **Find Your BALANCE** recommendations the day before and the day after the event.
- ❏ Book in some physical activity (i.e. tubing, a hike) earlier in the day of the event or the day after.
- ❏ Have your child plan the choices she is going to make (i.e. what she really wants to eat and what she can pass on) and write these down.

Once you have helped your child come up with a game plan that does not have her at cross purposes with important objectives, then you can move on to other steps in the family meeting such as role playing and affirmation.

Most of the time family meetings turn out very well. One of the primary reasons is because of the type of preparation and support shown in the Christmas holiday example. Parents find they are empowering their child to feel more in control of a situation that leaves many people feeling helpless. With a *Kids in Balance* game plan firmly in hand and both parental and *KIB* material support, you will likely be very encouraged by most of the choices your child makes over the next few months. There will also, however, be occasions when your child chooses to go off the *KIB* program and will need discussion and strategies as to how to get back on track. In either scenario, family meetings are the setting where your child can deepen her sense of belief in her own ability to make healthy choices. That is one of the best gifts, Christmas or otherwise, that you can give your child.

Family Communication Activity—An Example

What	How
Purpose	❑ Help family members deal with a difficult situation.
Equipment	❑ All family members. ❑ A parent as facilitator/leader.
Directions	❑ Explain the purpose of the meeting (i.e. to discuss health goals in relation to an upcoming Christmas season). ❑ Start with positive recognition (i.e. mention specific achievements each member has made in the recent past and let them know how proud you are of them). ❑ Outline the agenda item more specifically (i.e. describe the special event challenges that are upcoming). ❑ Ask for input (i.e. some may feel they will miss out if they stick to the *KIB* game plan, some may feel like parents will nag). ❑ Give your own input (i.e. you may want your family to celebrate without compromising good health; you may not want to feel like you worked hard for nothing, which would happen if you go to the work of providing healthy food choices over Christmas and family members make unhealthy choices anyway; you may really want to see your family enjoy themselves). ❑ Have family members express their goal(s) with regard to the agenda item. (i.e. continue to eat 7 servings of vegetables/day; to increase Sometimes Foods servings to 1/day; to have one event where they do not have to think about the *KIB* approach). ❑ List each member's goals on a piece of paper or flip chart. ❑ Strategize ways to achieve the various objectives (i.e. discussion around goals and desires until there is agreement on the level of effort that will at least maintain current achievement). ❑ Role-play any potential situations (i.e. a friend offering additional Sometime Food choices beyond what your child has agreed upon) and help your child determine a response. ❑ Come to family agreement as to how the particular agenda item will be handled and affirm family members as to a job well done (i.e. before the event, your child will let you know if she requires any substitute foods; you will provide the foods then will leave her alone to enjoy her evening). Congratulate your family on doing an amazing job of redefining the holiday season.

Appendix 7

Worksheets

Worksheets are helpful tools to assist you in reaching your *Kids in Balance* goals. They are either handy reference as you begin your wellness journey (i.e. *Natural Sweeteners* and *Kitchen Substitutes*) or useful templates that can be photocopied from the book or downloaded and printed from the *Kids in Balance* site at www.kidsinbalance.net/kib-resources-1.html.

Use the worksheets to keep track of any correlation between food, moods and activity levels, to help in goal setting and as handy templates for meal planning and grocery shopping.

While the completion of most of the worksheets is self-explanatory or is clearly outlined previously in the book, for two charts, please note the following additional information.

For the *Food, Mood, Activity Log*, and the *How Am I Doing? Chart*, print out a copy for each day they are needed, or put the chart in a plastic sleeve and use a non-permanent felt marker to tick off or fill in the appropriate squares that will show through the sleeve. As well, with both worksheets plan regular reviews. Each night, go over the log and/or chart with your child, strategize for the next day and then wipe the sleeve clean and re-use. Focus on specific conclusions or goals noted on the log or chart; during discussion of the worksheets use language that builds up; and while it is important to talk about areas that need improvement, be sure to also note what is already being done well.

Worksheet 1 - *Food, Mood, Activity Log*

As you and your child keep track of daily food intake, activity (i.e. physical exertion, screen time) and mood shifts throughout the day, you will begin to better understand your child's unique and natural responses to different types of food and activities. The conclusions you draw (i.e. high sugar-content cookie intake leads to fatigue, excessive computer time contributes to irritation, calmness comes after a snack of nuts and an apple) will help you gain insight that allows your child to take better control of food and activity choices. That insight, in turn, can provide increased likelihood of your child reaching her health and wellness goals.

Be sure to evaluate mood based on a wide range of criteria that includes descriptions such as: low or blue, cranky, irritable, bored, brain-fogged, enthusiastic, optimistic, thankful, calm and cheery. It can also be helpful to include physical responses such as bloating, headaches, energetic, strong, tired or weak.

Worksheet 10 - *How Am I Doing? Chart*

At the designated times in the *KIB* program, have your child complete the *How Am I Doing? Chart*. An easy way for your child to keep track of how she is keeping her body in balance is to add up the check marks in the Reaching my Goals column of the *How Am I Doing? Chart* and then subtract from that number, the amount of check marks in the Not There Yet column. The goal is to have the resulting sum be a number that increases over time. That means your child would be having an increasing number of check marks in the Reaching my Goals column and a decreasing number of check marks in the Not There Yet column.

Worksheet 1—*Food/Mood/Activity Log*

Meal	Mood Before	Food/Drink Intake	Mood After	Conclusion
Breakfast				
Snack				
Lunch				
Snack				
Dinner				
Snack				
Time	Mood Before	Type of Activity	Mood After	Conclusion
Morning				
Afternoon				
Evening				

Worksheet 2 — *Measure-up Chart*

KIB Measure-up Chart for:											
Date:											
Upper arm											
Lower arm											
Chest											
Waist											
Hips											
Thighs											
Calves											
Height											
Weight											
WHtR - Waist Divided by Height											

Worksheet 3—*Finding Your Motivators*

How I Have Felt Up Until Now	How I will Feel After I Succeed in Finding a Healthier Balance for my Body
Describe a time when your excess weight made you feel really sad . . .	Describe how you will feel when you lose unnecessary excess weight . . .
Describe a time when your excess weight made you feel embarrassed . . .	Looking at the times when your weight made you feel sad or embarrassed, describe how those situations would be different without the excess weight . . .
List some things that you do that are more difficult because of your extra weight . . .	List some things that would be easier for you to do without the extra weight . . .
Finish this sentence: "If you really knew me, you would know that I feel this about my body . . ."	Describe how you will feel about your body when you are not carrying this extra weight . . .

Worksheet 4—*Setting Your Goals*

When	How
Days 1-7 **Preparation Week**	Goal: Motivator:
Days 1-7 **Find Your BALANCE**	Goal: Motivator:
Days 8-14 **Find Your BALANCE**	Goal: Motivator:
Days 15-21 **Find Your BALANCE**	Goal: Motivator:
Every week of Build Your BALANCE	Goal: Motivator:
6 Months Into Build Your BALANCE	Goal: Motivator:
9 Months Into Build Your BALANCE	Goal: Motivator:
Upon Reaching Keep Your BALANCE	Goal: Motivator:

Setting Your Goals–An Example

When	How
Days 1-7 **Preparation Week**	**Goal**: Read *Day-at-a-Glance Guidelines* and do preparation week homework at least 5 days this week. **Motivator**: A family games night where I get to choose the game.
Days 1-7 **Find Your BALANCE**	**Goal**: Increase my vegetable intake by one serving each day. **Motivator**: Get an "excused from Saturday chore list" reward.
Days 8-14 **Find Your BALANCE**	**Goal**: Spend 10 minutes jumping on the trampoline at least 6 days this week. **Motivator**: A copy of my favourite magazine.
Days 15-21 **Find Your BALANCE**	**Goal**: Follow **Find Your BALANCE** *Day-at-a-Glance Guidelines* 6 out of 7 days this week. **Motivator**: Get to pick favourite new *KIB* recipe for supper—complete with helium balloons and congratulation speech!
Every week of Build Your BALANCE	**Goal**: Stick to **Build Your BALANCE** food list 6 out of 7 days a week. **Motivator**: $10 a week put into savings account toward a new wardrobe.
6 Months Into Build Your BALANCE	**Goal**: Do PACE interval training for 15 minutes/day, 3 days a week for 6 months. **Motivator**: Dad and mom contribute a pro-rated amount each week the goal is met; the money is saved to match what I contribute toward purchase of a bike.
9 Months Into Build Your BALANCE	**Goal**: Eat per *KIB* **Build Your BALANCE** with only 3 Sometimes Foods per week for 9 months. **Motivator**: Each week goal is met, a pro-rated amount is put toward a pedicure, manicure and updo hairstyle for graduation.
Upon Reaching Keep Your BALANCE	**Goal**: Move into healthy weight range; **Keep Your BALANCE** reached. **Motivator**: Clothes shopping trip with mom with saving account money.

Worksheet 5—*Kitchen Substitutes*[1]

During the first week of **Find Your BALANCE**, you will begin to transition from foods that are part of a Standard North American Diet to foods that are Eat for Health choices. As you gradually reduce refined sugars and grains, unhealthy oils, and processed foods, the list below will give suggestions as to what substitutes can replace former pantry choices. Not all of the Eat for Health foods listed below will be used during **Find Your BALANCE**, but eventually they will all be gradually added back into your dietary plan during **Build Your BALANCE** and **Keep Your BALANCE**.

Less healthy foods to transition from	*KIB* Eat for Health foods to substitute
White flours	Whole grain flours (i.e. wheat, rye, spelt)
Processed, sugar-sweetened cereals	Whole grain, high fibre, low sugar cereals
White rice and pastas	Brown or basmati rice, barley, whole grain pasta
Sugar sweetened jam	Fruit juice sweetened jam or bananas on toast
Soda pop	Filtered water or sparkling water with juice
Sugar-sweetened fruit juices, drinks	No sugar added fruit juices in small amounts
Margarine	Butter for taste and flavour
Shortening, palm, corn, canola oils	Olive oil, coconut oil, nut oils, sunflower oil
Coffee	Organic, fair-trade coffee (avoid for children)
Black tea	Green tea, rooibos tea (limit green tea with children)
Peanut butter with added sugar	Peanuts only peanut butter or other nut butters
Canned fruit	Fresh fruit in moderation
Canned/packaged soups	Homemade soup
Packaged cookies	Homemade cookies
Table salt	Sea salt, spices, Spike, Herbamare
White bread	Whole grain bread, whole grain sprouted bread, gluten-free bread
Potato chips, junk food snacks	Homemade nut and seed trail mix, hummus
Regular eggs	Free-range eggs
Farmed salmon	Wild salmon
Flavoured, sweetened yogurt	Plain yogurt (add fresh fruit if desired)
White/brown sugar, pancake syrup	Stevia, honey, maple syrup, evaporated cane juice, palm and date sugars
Artificial sweeteners–Splenda, Sugar Twin, Aspartame, Acesulfame K	Stevia, honey, maple syrup, evaporated cane juice, palm and date sugars

Worksheet 6—*Healthy Foods List (Find Your BALANCE)*[1]

Meat, Eggs	Vegetables	Nuts & Seeds	Beans & Legumes
Beef	Artichoke	Almonds	Black beans
Bison	Asparagus	Brazil nuts	Black-eyed peas
Chicken	Avocado	Cashews	Chickpeas
Cornish hen	Broccoli	Chia and salba seeds	Kidney beans
Duck	Brussels sprouts	Filberts (hazelnuts)	Lentils
Eggs	Cabbage	Flax seeds	Pinto beans
Elk	Carrots	Hemp seeds	Romano beans
Goose	Cauliflower	Hickory nuts	Snap peas
Lamb	Celery	Macadamia nuts	Snow peas
Moose	Cucumber	Peanuts	Split peas
Pork (in moderation)	Eggplant	Pecans	White (navy) beans
Rabbit	Green beans	Pine nuts	**Condiments & Misc.**
Turkey	Lettuces	Pistachios	Apple cider vinegar
Venison	Leeks	Pumpkin seeds	(unpasteurized)
Fish & Seafood*	Mushrooms	Sesame seeds	Balsamic vinegar
Crab (in moderation)	Olives	Sunflower seeds	Carob powder
Lobster (in moderation)	Onions	Walnuts	Cocoa powder
Prawns (in moderation)	Peppers	**Nut Butters**	Coconut milk
Scallop (in moderation)	Radishes	Almond butter	Dijon mustard
Shrimp (in moderation)	Rutabaga	Peanut butter	(unsweetened)
Wild fish	Scallions	**Fats & Oils**	Flavour extracts
Dairy	Shallots	Butter	(real, not artificial)
Kefir (unsweetened)	Spinach	Coconut oil	Garlic
Medium fat cheeses	Sprouts	Flaxseed oil	Herbs (fresh, dried)
(not skim, low or full)	Swiss chard	(cold pressed)	Mayonnaise
Organic cheeses	(and other greens)	Olive oil	(unsweetened)
European cheeses	Tomato	(extra virgin, virgin)	Protein powder
(i.e. Gouda, Jarlsberg)	Turnip	Safflower oil	(whey, hemp)
Plain yogurt	Zucchini [courgette]	Sesame oil	Salsa (unsweetened)
(unsweetened)	(and other squashes)	Sunflower oil	Sea salt
Fruit	**Sweeteners**	**Beverages**	Soy (tofu, tempeh)
Cranberries	Stevia	Herbal teas	(organic, fermented)
Lemon	Xylitol	Vegetable juice	
Lime		Water (filtered)	

* For smart and sustainable choices when eating seafood, visit: www.oceansalive.org.

Worksheet 7—Weekly Menu Plan Template

Meal	Day 1	Day 2	Day 3	Day 4	Day 5	Day 6	Day 7
Breakfast							
Snack							
Lunch							
Snack							
Dinner							
Snack							

Worksheet 8—*Portion Size Guidelines*

This Zimbabwe measurement method, suggested by Dr K Mawji, illustrates how to use one's hand to measure food portions simply, imaginatively and in a reasonably accurate manner.

Shown below with illustrations and explanations adapted by the Canadian Diabetes Association, the guidelines are an easy tool to teach your child appropriate portion sizes. And as your child's hands will grow as he grows, the Handy Portion Guide is a tool that will, for the most part, be a guideline that will serve him well for life.

During **Build Your BALANCE** and for Protein Body Types during **Keep Your BALANCE**, however, your child may need to choose an amount of fruits/grains and starches that is ½ the size of his fist instead of the recommended full fist size. Take a look again at the information on *Fuel Mix Guidelines* and the *Fuel Mix Evaluation Chart* to ensure your child is experiencing the benefits of a correct fuel mix for his unique metabolism

If your child does not have dairy allergies or intolerances, you can include dairy products as part of his daily protein intake. If possible, however, find an organic source, and if your child is young or is a Protein Body Type, ensure the milk contains at least 2% fat.

Handy portion guide

Your hands can be very useful in estimating appropriate portions. When planning a meal, use the following portion sizes as a guide:

 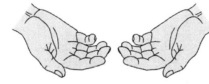 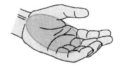

FRUITS*/GRAINS & STARCHES*:
Choose an amount the size of your fist for each of Grains &Starches, and Fruit.

VEGETABLES*:
Choose as much as you can hold in both hands.

MEAT & ALTERNATIVES*:
Choose an amount up to the size of the palm of your hand and the thickness of your little finger.

FATS*:
Limit fat to an amount the size of the tip of your thumb.

MILK & ALTERNATIVES*: Drink up to 250 mL (8 oz) of low-fat milk with a meal.

* Food group names taken from Beyond the Basics: Meal Planning for Healthy Eating, Diabetes Prevention and Management © Canadian Diabetes Association, 2005. Please refer to this resource for more details on meal planning.

Sweetener	Uses	Substitutions
Stevia (from a shrub of the astor family), **Lou Han Guo** (fruit extract) and **Xylitol**. Main *KIB*-friendly sweeteners—especially during **Find Your BALANCE**.	Stevia—all types of cooking, beverages (adjust ratio of wet ingredients to dry ingredients) Lou han guo—usually processed into a powder; good in all types of cooking/baking	Stevia—depending upon form, 8-300 times sweeter than sugar. Use in powdered or liquid form and follow directions on container for substitution recommendations. Lou han guo—low-glycemic and roughly 200 times sweeter than sugar. Use per package directions. Xylitol—generally found in some manufactured products.
Unpasteurized Honey (This form has nutrient-rich substances still available. Do not serve honey to children under the age of two because of potential for botulism).	Baked goods, herbal teas, drizzled on tart fruit	20-60 times sweeter than sugar. Substitute ½ to ¾ cup (125 to 190 ml) for 1 cup (250 ml) white sugar. Reduce liquid by ¼ cup (60 ml), or add 3-4 extra tablespoons of flour. Add ¼ tsp (1 ml) baking soda per 1 cup (250 ml) honey. Reduce oven temperature by 25 degrees and adjust baking time as edges of baked goods can brown quickly.
Brown rice syrup or **barley malt syrup**	Baked goods (i.e. spice cakes), homemade granola, baked beans	For cakes, combine with another sweetener such as maple syrup. Substitute 1⅓ cups (325 ml) for 1 cup (250 ml) white sugar. Reduce liquid by ¼ cup (60 ml), or add 3-4 extra tablespoons of flour. Add ¼ tsp (1 ml) baking soda per 1 cup (250 ml) rice syrup.
Agave syrup or **nectar** (Produced in Mexico from the agave plant; controversial because of high fructose content and ultra-refinement with most brands. Ensure organic, high quality sources).	Baked goods, salad dressings, hot or cold beverages (dissolves in hot or cold liquids)	Substitute ⅓ cup (80 ml) for 1 cup (250 ml) white sugar. Reduce liquid by ¼ cup (60 ml), or add 3-4 extra tablespoons flour. Reduce oven temperature by 25 degrees and adjust baking time. Because of high fructose content, best to use minimally.
Evaporated cane juice (i.e. Sucanat, Panela brands) is sugar cane with fibre and water removed. Read labels well to ensure it is simply evaporated cane syrup.	Baked goods, tea	Substitute ⅔ to ¾ cup (165 to 190 ml) for 1 cup (250 ml) white sugar.
Palm sugar, coconut sugar and date sugar (less commonly found sugars made from the sap of palm trees, coconut trees and dates).	Baked goods, general all-purpose sweeteners (Note: date sugar does not dissolve well in hot beverages)	Generally lower glycemic and with higher nutrient levels; look for organic or pure forms (i.e. not cut with sucrose) and substitute in equal amounts as white sugar.
Unsulphured blackstrap molasses	Pumpkin or zucchini [courgette] loaf, muffins, cookies	Great sweetener for muffins or loaves. Substitute in equal amounts as white sugar, but combine with other sweeteners, as taste is strong.
Pure maple syrup	Baked goods, cakes, puddings	Substitute ⅔ to ¾ cup (165 to 190 ml) maple syrup for 1 cup (250 ml) white sugar. Reduce liquid by 3 tablespoons (45 ml). Also add ¼ tsp (1 ml) baking soda per 1 cup (250 ml) maple syrup.

Worksheet 10 – *How Am I Doing? Chart*

B-A-L-A-N-C-E	Reaching my Goals	Not There Yet
B - Body type	Carb ☐ Protein ☐ Mixed ☐	Don't know ☐
A - Attitude	Think you can! ☐	Think you can't. ☐
L - Laughter	5-10 good laughs ☐	0-4 good laughs ☐
A – Activity (☐= 15 minute increments)	Physical Activity ☐ ☐ ☐ ☐ ☐ ☐ ☐ ☐ ☐	Screen ☐ ☐ ☐ ☐ ☐ ☐ ☐ ☐ ☐
N – a good Night's sleep	Goal met ☐	Goal not met ☐
C – Clean water (check ☐ for extra cups)	4 cups (8 oz/250ml each) ☐ ☐ ☐ ☐ ☐ ☐	< 4 cups (8 oz/250ml each) ☐ Pop, sugary juice ☐ ☐ ☐
E – Eat for health	Balanced (Fuel Mix, Food Pairing, Comfortable Fullness)	Unbalanced (wrong Fuel Mix, too much or not enough food)
Breakfast	☐	☐
Snack	☐	☐
Lunch	☐	☐
Snack	☐	☐
Dinner	☐	☐
Snack	☐	☐
Sometimes Foods	None ☐	☐ ☐ ☐ ☐ ☐
Important *KIB* "Extras"		
Bowel movements	☐ ☐ ☐	<1 ☐
Hugs or "I love you"s given and received.	☐ ☐ ☐ ☐ ☐	<1 ☐
1_____ - 2 _____ = Total _____	Column 1 checks =	Column 2 checks =

Worksheet 11–*Healthy Foods List (Build Your BALANCE and Keep Your BALANCE)*[1]

Meat & Eggs	Vegetables	Nuts & Seeds	Beans & Legumes
Beef	Artichoke	Almonds	Black beans
Bison	Asparagus	Brazil nuts	Black-eyed peas
Chicken	Avocado	Cashews	Chickpeas
Cornish hen	Beets	Chia and salba seeds	Kidney beans
Duck	Broccoli	Filberts (hazelnuts)	Lentils
Eggs	Brussels sprouts	Flax seeds	Pinto beans
Elk	Cabbage	Hemp seeds	Snap peas
Goose	Carrots	Hickory nuts	Snow peas
Lamb	Cauliflower	Macadamia nuts	Split peas
Moose	Celery	Peanuts	White (navy) beans
Pork (in moderation)	Corn	Pecans	**Nut Butters**
Rabbit	Cucumber	Pine nuts	Almond butter
Turkey	Eggplant	Pistachios	Cashew butter
Venison	Green beans	Pumpkin seeds	Peanut butter
Fish & Seafood*	Lettuces	Sesame seeds	**Condiments & Misc.**
Crab (in moderation)	Leeks	Sunflower seeds	Apple cider vinegar
Lobster (in moderation)	Mushrooms	Walnuts	(unpasteurized)
Prawns (in moderation)	Olives	**Fats & Oils**	Balsamic vinegar
Scallop (in moderation)	Onions	Butter	Carob powder
Shrimp (in moderation)	Peppers	Coconut oil	Cocoa powder
Wild fish	Potato	Flaxseed oil	Coconut milk
Dairy	Radishes	(cold pressed)	Dijon mustard
Kefir (unsweetened)	Rutabaga	Olive oil	(unsweetened)
Medium fat cheeses	Scallions	(extra virgin, virgin)	Flavour extracts
(not skim, low or full)	Shallots	Safflower oil	(real, not artificial)
Organic cheeses	Spinach	Sesame oil	Garlic
European cheeses	Sprouts	Sunflower oil	Herbs (fresh, dried)
(i.e. Gouda, Jarlsberg)	Sweet potato, yam	**Fruit**	Mayonnaise
Plain yogurt	Swiss chard	Apples	(unsweetened)
(unsweetened)	(and other greens)	Apricots	Protein powder
Grains (if tolerated)	Tomato	Berries	(whey, hemp)
Barley	Turnip	Cherries	Salsa (unsweetened)
Quinoa	Zucchini [courgette]	Citrus fruit	Sea salt
Rice (basmati, wild)	(and other squashes)	Kiwi	Soy (tofu, tempeh)
Rolled oats	**Sweeteners**	Mangoes	(organic, fermented)
(not instant)	Honey	Melons	**Beverages**
Whole grain bread	Molasses	Peaches	Fruit juice (limited)
(sprouted, if possible)	Stevia	Pears	Herbal teas
Whole grain crackers	Unrefined cane sugar	Pineapple	Vegetable juice
(rice, rye, wheat)	Xylitol	Plums	Water (filtered)

* For smart and sustainable choices when eating seafood, visit: www.oceansalive.org.

Appendix 8

Day-at-a-Glance Guidelines
Find Your BALANCE

Moving your child through a week of preparation and then onto **Find Your BALANCE** is straightforward and simple. Because the *KIB* program covers a range of factors that contribute to excess weight, however, accounting for each of those BALANCE factors—**B**ody type, **A**ttitude, **L**aughter and play, **A**ctivity, a good **N**ight's sleep, **C**lean water and **E**at for health—can sometimes make simple seem a little complex.

That's why the *KIB Day-at-a-Glance Guidelines* were created. For each of your seven days of preparation and your three weeks of **Find Your BALANCE**, you will have a sheet that outlines daily actions in each of the BALANCE areas. Photocopy the *Day-at-a-Glance Guidelines* from this book, or go to www.kidsinbalance.net/kib-resources-1.html to download and print the guidelines from there.

Every night, simply take a look at the actions required for the following day, check your day timer or calendar to see where to best fit in those simple activities and easily take the next small step toward increasing your child's health and wellness.

Preparation Week

In the week of preparation before **Find Your BALANCE** begins, there is **no change in diet or activity levels**. Though this week may seem somewhat inactive it is actually crucial to the success of the program. Rather than tackling a series of new tasks each day, you are simply recording your child's/family's current state and beginning the mental and physical preparation for the three weeks of **Find Your BALANCE**. Knowing where you are with your lifestyle choices and the results those choices have produced can be a powerful motivator for change.

Find Your BALANCE - Week One

In the first week of **Find Your BALANCE**, you and your child will begin to make small changes in each of *KIB*'s seven solution areas, and by the end of that week, will be more familiar with the seven factors that will contribute to your child reaching a healthy weight—**B**ody type, **A**ttitude, **L**aughter and play, **A**ctivity, a good **N**ight's sleep, **C**lean water and **E**at for health. These small steps will make it easier for you to transition to the final two weeks of **Find Your BALANCE** where the dietary and lifestyle changes will be more extensive and intensive.

Find Your BALANCE - Weeks Three and Four

After completing both a week of preparation and week one of **Find Your BALANCE**, your family should now be ready to tackle the final two weeks of this phase which include a much more structured dietary and lifestyle plan. Along with your final two weeks of *Day-at-a-Glance Guidelines*, you will need a two-week menu plan (either *KIB*'s sample *Find Your BALANCE Menu Plans* that can be found at www.kidsinbalance.net/kib-resources-1.html or your own version of the

Find Your BALANCE menu plans) and a shopping list. Making good use of this phase's, *Day-at-a-Glance Guidelines* gives you a strong foundation for finishing up **Find Your BALANCE** in a positive and beneficial way. Ensure you have answered chapter 10's "Twenty Questions to Ask Yourself Before You Begin **Find Your BALANCE**" (p. 79) with a resounding "yes," and if so, go for it!

Congratulations! The beginning of your *KIB* journey starts today.

Day-at-a-Glance Guidelines
Preparation Week—Day 1

TIP of the day:

Mark today as the start of a journey. Begin "x" ing the family calendar or better yet, head for the local high school race track and take a photo of family members all lined up in start position at the beginning of a lap!

What's On the Menu?

Food Formula: continue eating as normal

Managing the Day

B - Body Type: Over the next number of weeks you will be learning more about body type and how it impacts optimal food choice. Today begin to look and see the different sizes and shapes of bodies around you in your family, school and community.

A - Attitude: Take 10-15 minutes during the day to ask how everyone is feeling about the adventure you are starting. Acknowledge the range of emotions (i.e. fear, excitement, apprehension) and help each other determine what lies beneath the emotion (i.e. concern because of loss of familiar food items or that you will be hungry, worry that weight loss will impact relationship with friends). Look at the information on language that builds up (p. 41) and, if need be, help each other re-frame concerns positively.

L - Laughter/Play: Find out the funniest thing that happened to each family member during the past week.

A - Activity: Maintain normal amounts of physical activity and screen time. Along with daily food intake and moods, record that activity and screen time on *KIB's Food/Mood/Activity Log*.

N - Night's Sleep: On your *Food/Mood/Activity Log*, record how many hours of sleep your child had.

C - Clean Water: Take note of how many glasses of water each family member drank today.

E - Eat for Health: Food logs are an essential component of the *KIB* program. They help determine both types of foods eaten and food patterns (i.e. when in a day foods are eaten) and give crucial clues as to what shifts in food choices and eating times need to be made to ensure optimum health. For more information take a look at chapter 10's Food Logs: Why *KIB* Loves Them.

Day-at-a-Glance Guidelines
Preparation Week—Day 2

TIP of the day:

If you have a busy schedule, you may not get all today's homework done. While prioritizing KIB activities is key to making the program work, if today was hectic, be sure that at least the food log and measurement chart get completed.

What's On the Menu?

Food Formula: continue eating as normal

Managing the Day

B - Body Type: Observe how many of your family members are shorter and rounder, and how many are taller and leaner. Consider grandparents and aunts and uncles on each side of the family too. Do you see some patterns in shape/size?

A - Attitude: Take your child's measurements per *KIB's Measure-up Chart* (p. 212) and do a weigh-in. If this is difficult for your child, talk about what makes the reality check a hard activity. Remember that numbers do not determine who a person is, but they are helpful tools to see if there is need for healthful change.

L - Laughter/Play: Make time for a short family activity (i.e. bedtime reading, quick game of cards or a round of bocce).

A - Activity: Maintain normal amounts of physical activity and screen time. Along with daily food intake and moods, record that activity and screen time on *KIB's Food/Mood/Activity Log*.

N - Night's Sleep: Continue to record hours of sleep each night.

C - Clean Water: Again check the amount of water each family member drank today. Are there family members who do not drink much water? Find out why (i.e. taste, forgetfulness, convenience).

E - Eat for Health: Take a look at your first day's *Food/Mood/Activity Log*. Circle foods that contain refined grains or sugars. Draw a square around protein foods and a triangle around vegetables. Not sure which foods are which? Check out chapter 9 - **Eat for Health**.

Day-at-a-Glance Guidelines
Preparation Week — Day 3

TIP of the day:

Talking about the experiences and feelings excess weight promotes can be difficult. Start the conversations in places your child feels safe. Some suggestions are: in a quiet time before bed, driving in the car or around the family table.

What's On the Menu?

Food Formula: continue eating as normal

Managing the Day

B - Body Type: Sometimes simple details give clues to body type. Check family members' ear lobes. Often longer or larger ear lobes can be a characteristic of Protein Body Types. Compare type of ear lobes with the results on the *KIB Body Type Survey* and see how accurately the two match up.

A - Attitude: Begin a goals and motivators discussion with your child. Follow the format in *KIB*'s *Finding Your Motivators* worksheet (p. 213) and talk about experiences and feelings your child has had up until now with regard to excess weight. Next look at the types of feelings or experiences that will be possible once your child is in a healthy weight range. Finally, using *KIB*'s *Setting Your Goals* worksheet and the goals and desires information in chapter 4, begin to discuss the types of goals you and your child want to put into place. Continue this discussion over the next few days as you and your child plan a healthy variety of internal and external goals and motivators.

L - Laughter/Play: Have family members share their funniest or most embarrassing moment.

A - Activity: Maintain normal amounts of physical activity and screen time. Record activity and screen time, along with food intake and mood, on *KIB*'s *Food/Mood/Activity Log*.

N - Night's Sleep: Continue to record hours of sleep each night and your child's bedtime.

C - Clean Water: Did you know that almost 70% of your body is composed of water? See how many glasses you drank today to replenish that volume.

E - Eat for Health: What is in our kitchen is often a good indication of the health of our bodies. Have your child list the varieties of fruits and vegetables in your kitchen, or if shopping day is just around the corner—and your fridge, freezer and kitchen cupboards are pretty empty—have the list reflect what is usually in your kitchen.

Day-at-a-Glance Guidelines
Preparation Week—Day 4

> **TIP of the day:**
> *Have parents (or even call and have grandparents) share about the types of food they ate as children and the types of activity they did. Remember though: no one ever walked up hill both back and forth to school!*

What's On the Menu?

Food Formula: continue eating as normal

Managing the Day

B - Body Type: If your kids have recently studied the diet of the North American Inuit people group in school, have them share their discoveries. If not, do a book or online search and record your findings. Compare this type of diet to the diet of people living in Northern India.

A - Attitude: Take several photos of your child. Include full-length photos as well as close-ups. Sometimes photo taking can be a difficult activity as children may have begun to experience some embarrassment over the excess weight they carry. Continue to use language that builds up to help your child understand that excess weight is not who they are. Photos are simply a way of recording where your child is with regard to a healthy balanced weight and therefore will be a good way for your child to see positive change as he begins making healthier lifestyle choices.

L - Laughter/Play: Designate one family member as the joke teller for the day. If his or her repertoire is pretty slim, check online resources for family jokes and wow other family members with the comedy routine.

A - Activity: Maintain normal amounts of physical activity and screen time. Record activity and screen time, along with food intake and mood, on *KIB's Food/Mood/Activity Log.*

N - Night's Sleep: What time do family members get up and do they wake rested?

C - Clean Water: If we are drinking enough water, our urine is usually light-coloured or clear. Ask family members to take note of the colour of their urine and then record the colors. After a couple of weeks you can do this exercise again and compare results.

E - Eat for Health: Take a look at the past three days' *Food/Mood/Activity Logs.* On average, how many and what type of beverages does each family member consume each day?

Day-at-a-Glance Guidelines
Preparation Week—Day 5

> **TIP of the day:**
> *When talking about favourite foods and flavours remember you are brainstorming and sharing ideas. Everyone's ideas, even if they seem to be nutritionally poor choices, are still valid and can serve as starting points for recipes to later adapt.*

What's On the Menu?

Food Formula: continue eating as normal

Managing the Day

B - Body Type: Find out which family members like physical activity and if they like doing activity by themselves (i.e. walking alone or working out by themselves) or if they prefer activity that is done in groups (i.e. playing ball hockey, a dance class). Often Protein Body Types do not prefer physical activity but will participate if it can be done in groups where there can be social interaction or a team effort. Carbohydrate Body Types tend to enjoy exercise, both individually and in groups.

A - Attitude: Continue discussion around goals and motivators. Ask questions such as "What makes you happy?" or "What bring you peace?" to explore the types of motivators that bring longer lasting satisfaction. Do not, however, minimize motivators that are more short term. Choosing a new t-shirt as a reward for consistently making healthy food choices can be a fine goal. Remember to avoid the use of poor quality Sometimes Foods for motivators. They do not help your wellness cause.

L - Laughter/Play: Make time for a family walk. Even a 10-minute walk around the block counts! Take note of what is new (i.e. spring buds, leaves turning colour, a neighbour's car).

A - Activity: Maintain normal amounts of physical activity and screen time. Record activity and screen time, along with food intake and mood, on *KIB's Food/Mood/Activity Log.*

N - Night's Sleep: If you have trouble falling asleep some nights, see if you can discover any link between that particular sleep challenge and the type of foods eaten late in the day.

C - Clean Water: If water intake is low, start upping your child's water levels days 8-14 of **Find Your BALANCE**. Some tips: add lemon slices, or get a new water bottle (glass or stainless steel).

E - Eat for Health: Have your child talk about favorite foods and flavours. Next week you will be discovering ways to make some of those familiar foods and flavours work for **Find Your BALANCE.**

Day-at-a-Glance Guidelines
Preparation Week—Day 6

TIP of the day:
Be sure everyone gets in several good belly laughs today, even if you have to resort to tickling or parental "groaner" jokes.

What's On the Menu?

Food Formula: continue eating as normal

Managing the Day

B - Body Type: Ask family members how they like to organize their rooms. If they like things very orderly (i.e. clothes organized by colour or type, bookshelves neat and tidy) it is often indicative of a Carbohydrate Body Type. Protein Body Types tend to organize in a different way. Even when cleaned, their rooms can often look quite untidy, but they generally know where the item they are looking for is tucked away. Mixed Body Types often use a combination of organizational styles.

A - Attitude: How are family members feeling about the changes that will begin next week? Encourage each other to think positively about the new ways you will be doing life.

L - Laughter/Play: Watch a funny TV show—*America's Funniest Home Videos* anyone?

A - Activity: Maintain normal amounts of physical activity and screen time. Record activity and screen time, along with food intake and mood, on *KIB's Food/Mood/Activity Log.*

N - Night's Sleep: The hours we sleep before midnight are extremely important. Teenagers can be tempted to stay up late playing games on the computer or instant messaging friends. Look at your sleep patterns and see if there are nights where you got little or no pre-midnight sleep time.

C - Clean Water: Think about the different ways you enjoy water (i.e. swimming, playing in the ocean, kayaking, summer water fights, soaking in a hot bath). Isn't it great that water is helpful both inside our body and outside our body?

E - Eat for Health: Take a look at the last five days of *Food/Mood/Activity Log*s. Note where the refined grains and sugars are showing up and talk about ways the family can gradually reduce those food types next week. Ideas would be to switch a two-cookie snack to a one-cookie snack or to have half as much pasta or rice for supper.

Day-at-a-Glance Guidelines
Preparation Week—Day 7

TIP of the day:

Through the day make a mental note of comments, dreams, hopes and requests your child mentions. Her words give good clues as to some potentially helpful motivators.

What's On the Menu?

Food Formula: continue eating as normal

Managing the Day

B - Body Type: Look at the types of breakfasts you had this past week and any mood changes you noted after eating. Are there differences in mood after you eat breakfasts that are mostly grains (i.e. cereals, bagels, toast, waffles) and after you eat breakfasts that contain more protein such as eggs, nuts, nut butters, bacon, cheese, sausages or legumes?

A - Attitude: How do different family members view a glass that is half filled with water? Do some experience discouragement or negativity as they focus on the part that has no water in it while others are still positive and glad for the water that is there? Talk about how different ways of looking at situations impact our feelings about those situations.

L - Laughter/Play: Pull out a family photo album. Reminiscing over last year's Halloween costumes or summer vacation activities usually brings joy to the spirit!

A - Activity: Maintain normal amounts of physical activity and screen time. Record activity and screen time, along with food intake and mood, on *KIB's Food/Mood/Activity Log*.

N - Night's Sleep: Do family members sleep in on weekends? We work best on regular routines. Try to be in bed before 11:00 (depending upon age, by 8:00, 9:00 or 10:00) and up by 7:00 each day.

C - Clean Water: Take note of where you have physical activity in the week. Do you increase your water intake before or during walking the dog, soccer practise or a yoga class?

E - Eat for Health: Have family members make a list of vegetables they enjoy eating and another list of vegetables they are prepared to try. Younger children can do the exercise with photos of vegetables cut out of the grocery store flyers. Give the lists to the family member who does the meal planning and writes the shopping list so she or he can ensure there is a good supply of well-liked and "willing to try" vegetables in the house.

Day-at-a-Glance Guidelines
Find Your BALANCE—Day 1

TIP of the day:

Last week you learned new information but made no change to your diet and activity levels. This week you will begin making slight diet and lifestyle changes Have candles at dinner to celebrate!

What's On the Menu?

Food Formula: begin to reduce the amount of Sometimes Foods per the **Eat for Health** homework below.

Managing the Day

B - Body Type: Recognize that though there are a range of factors that determine appetite, in general Protein Body Types need to eat a larger volume of food to feel satisfied while Carbohydrate Body Types tend to feel full on less food. As Protein Body Types learn *KIB*'s Food Pairing principle, however, they will be able to more wisely choose foods to provide Comfortable Fullness.

A - Attitude: Beginning to make tangible dietary changes can produce heightened emotions of both excitement and loss. Make room to discuss a full range of potential feelings.

L - Laughter/Play: Sun, rain, or snow, head to the playground and toss around a Frisbee. Even if your family is Frisbee-throwing challenged, you will still enjoy a few laughs.

A - Activity: If last week's *Food/Mood/Activity Log* shows your child averages more than an hour or two of screen time each day, it is time to begin gradually reducing that amount this week.

N - Night's Sleep: Ensure your child's room is totally dark at night. If not, get room-darkening blinds or in a pinch, place a dark sheet over existing window coverings.

C - Clean Water: Do a count of where your pre-*Kids in Balance* water intake stands.

E - Eat for Health: Take a look at last week's *Food/Mood/Activity Log* and draw a triangle around any non-starchy vegetables listed, draw a square around any protein listed, draw a circle around any grains or starchy vegetables listed, draw a heart around any fats listed, draw an oval around fruit and draw a diamond around Sometimes Foods like candy, chocolate, pop, cookies or chips. Look at the average amounts of Sometimes Foods listed per day (i.e. 3 cookies, 2 granola bars, 1 pop) and today eat Sometimes Foods at roughly the same time in the day but in smaller amounts.

Day-at-a-Glance Guidelines
Find Your BALANCE—Day 2

TIP of the day:

If family members are having trouble remembering to drink more water, have them fill a pitcher with the daily amount for their body size and keep it in plain view. They need to try and empty the pitcher by bedtime.

What's On the Menu?

Food Formula: continue to reduce Sometimes Foods and begin to increase water intake.

Managing the Day

B - Body Type: If you have a day planned with lots of activity, remember to give your child the right breakfast fuel mix for stamina. While Carbohydrate Body Types have long-lasting energy with whole grains and fruit, Protein Body Types need at least a small amount of meat, nuts, eggs or dairy to give them staying power.

A - Attitude: Do a quote search, either in the library or online, and have family members find one encouraging attitude quote they can write up on a sticky note and post in a prominent place to review during the latter part of **Find Your BALANCE**.

L - Laughter/Play: Spend time learning a new card or dice game this evening. If none of your family members has one to teach, do a quick search online or call a friend.

A - Activity: One good way to reduce TV time is to allot a certain number of hours per week for viewing time and have family members choose which shows they will watch. Pre-planning both TV and computer time prevents sitting on the couch or at the computer for long periods of time either channel or web surfing.

N - Night's Sleep: If your child sleeps with a night-light, try moving it out into the hallway. That way the pathway to the bathroom is well lit but your child's room stays dark.

C - Clean Water: As family members work toward increasing their daily water intake this week, make a note of where the water fountains are at school and work and be sure to walk past them and take a drink on a regular basis!

E - Eat for Health: Take a look at last week's beverage intake for family members. Reduce intake of any beverage other than water to ½ of last week's amount. Replace the intake of other beverages with additional water. This may take several days to achieve.

Day-at-a-Glance Guidelines
Find Your BALANCE—Day 3

TIP of the day:

Begin implementation of a "one taste" family guideline. As you introduce new vegetables and proteins, and indeed whole new recipes over the next few months and beyond, it is important that family members try at least a small taste each time.

What's On the Menu?

Food Formula: continue to reduce Sometimes Foods, and increase water and vegetable intake.

Managing the Day

B - Body Type: Because different body types can have more or less appreciation for different food flavours (i.e. sour, sweet, salty) and textures, the "one taste" guideline give family members a chance to experience new foods but also gives freedom to say "thanks, that's enough for now." After the taste, if your child does not prefer the foodstuff, she can leave the remainder of one type of food (i.e. zucchini) out of the dish (i.e. salad or stir-fry).

A - Attitude: Have a quick discussion with your child today on the difference between goals and desires. Be sure she understands that the types of goals you and she will set and work toward over the next few months need to be things that are within her ability to complete and do not require the uncertain co-operation of someone else, or even her own body.

L - Laughter/Play: Regular quiet times can also bring about a de-stressing effect. Before bedtime, have your child lay still, with eyes closed, and listen to 5-10 minutes of her favorite quieter music.

A - Activity: If you run errands today, park your vehicle farther away from your destination and get in a little extra walk time. Also take the time today or tomorrow to photocopy (p. 221) or download (www.kidsinbalance.net/kib-resources-1.html) the *How Am I Doing? Chart* for Day 8.

N - Night's Sleep: Soothing baths can be a helpful part of a relaxing bedtime routine for your child.

C - Clean Water: As you drink water today, think about a few of the ways water helps keep you healthy: carries nutrients to your cells and carries waste material away from your cells, strengthens your immune system and helps keep your bowels moving well.

E - Eat for Health: Take a look at the vegetable lists that family members compiled. Add a new vegetable from the lists into today's menu plan and work toward your child eating at least one vegetable serving at lunch and dinner and all snack times.

Day-at-a-Glance Guidelines
Find Your BALANCE—Day 4

TIP of the day:

Ridding the cupboards and refrigerator of old food favourites can be an emotional time. Remember to begin getting new tasty looking recipes and snacks ready to replace them.

What's On the Menu?

Food Formula: reduce refined sugars and grains; increase protein, vegetables and water.

Managing the Day

B - Body Type: Protein and Carbohydrate Body Types look at food differently. Protein Types, with their "live to eat" approach may have a harder time giving up comfort foods than their Carbohydrate Type "eat to live" family members. Have grace for each other!

A - Attitude: The rise of emotions (i.e. sadness, frustration, anger, joy, anxiety) is something we have little control over. How we respond to emotions, however, is well within our control. Help your child grow in understanding that he chooses his responses. To that end, you are welcome to repeat the attitude quote I remind myself of often: "Attitude is everything; choose a good one."

L - Laughter/Play: See which family member can make the funniest face. If you have a digital camera, record the results and put together a slide show.

A - Activity: Look in the garage or basement and see what types of equipment you can pull out for a quick burst of activity. A hula-hoop, jump rope or mini-football is a good start.

N - Night's Sleep: If your child has trouble falling asleep, be sure his bedtime snack contains carbohydrates **and** protein. The combination of carbohydrates (i.e. fruit, whole grains) and the amino acid tryptophan in the protein (i.e. nuts) allow the production of serotonin. In the dark, serotonin is converted to melatonin, a hormone that helps us feel sleepy.

C - Clean Water: Be sure that every time the family heads to the car to run errands or go on an outing, each family member has a water bottle close at hand.

E - Eat for Health: Box up any non-*KIB*-friendly pantry or cupboard foods and prepare to move them out of the house. If they have some nutritional value (i.e. tinned soups) give them to a local food bank, otherwise dump the food and recycle the packaging. Unsure of what to keep and what to give away? Make use of *KIB's Kitchen Substitutes*, *Natural Sweeteners* and *Healthy Foods List* worksheets (Appendix 7) for guidelines and support.

Day-at-a-Glance Guidelines
Find Your BALANCE—Day 5

> **TIP of the day:**
>
> *Get all family members to have a last minute check of the menu plan for next week. You want to ensure everyone knows what is coming and has mentally prepared for the changes.*

What's On the Menu?

Food Formula: reduce refined sugars and grains; increase protein, vegetables and water.

Managing the Day

B - Body Type: As you wind down your intake of Sometimes Foods, try to have much smaller portions of desserts and choose desserts that are more supportive of your body type: Protein Types do better on richer desserts such as cheesecake, while Carbohydrate Types tend to do better on desserts such as fruit pie or cookies.

A - Attitude: Read the motivation quotes family members discovered a couple of days ago. Need another great quote to post in a prominent place? "One of the greatest powers in the universe is individual power of choice. And the most powerful choices are positive choices."(Frederick Mann)

L - Laughter/Play: Almost everyone has heard that it takes the use of more muscles to frown than it does to smile, but who in your family know how **many** muscles it takes to both frown and smile? An Internet search shows there is much confusion as to the correct answer. What we do know is that with human beings, facial expressions are contagious. Therefore, start the day with the responses you want to get back!

A - Activity: For functional fitness consider practical activities your child already does (i.e. take out the garbage, walk to school) and be more purposeful about them (i.e. power walk the garbage to the bin or pump arms back and forth on the way to school).

N - Night's Sleep: Though *KIB* loves activity, try to keep more strenuous exercise approximately an hour away from bedtime as some children have difficulty falling asleep right after exercise.

C - Clean Water: Space water intake throughout the day. If your child drinks a lot of her daily intake at bedtime, her sleep could be disrupted by visits to the bathroom.

E - Eat for Health: By now your child should be including a small amount of protein and vegetables each time she eats (other than occasionally omitting vegetables at breakfast). Refined grains and sugars intake should be at bare minimum, and water intake far outweighing juice or pop intake.

Day-at-a-Glance Guidelines
Find Your BALANCE—Day 6

> **TIP of the day:**
>
> *The word breakfast comes from the term "breaking the fast". By breakfast, a lot of time has gone by without eating and it is important to re-fuel with foods that support body type.*

What's On the Menu?

Food Formula: continue with previous dietary modifications and increase fitness.

Managing the Day

B - Body Type: Though Carbohydrate or Mixed Body Types may not be as hungry as Protein Body Types at breakfast, each family member needs to re-fuel. Ensure Protein Types get more protein than grains or fruit, along with fat, and that other family members include a higher percentage of grains and fruit than protein, and a little less fat.

A - Attitude: During days 8-21 of **Find Your BALANCE**, your child's moods may vary from excitement and joy to discouragement and sadness. Talk to him about the range of emotions that may be experienced and come up with some positive ways to handle each possibility.

L - Laughter/Play: Children often have a spontaneous side to their character. Part of a parent's job is to help a child become organized and able to handle the roles he will need to get along in the world. Be sure, however, to nurture your child's unprompted, spur-of-the-moment traits as well.

A - Activity: As you continue to increase functional fitness over the next few days, ensure there are a few group activities (i.e. bike rides, croquet tournament, a hike with friends) that meet the socializing component of activity that Protein Body Types often desire.

N - Night's Sleep: If your child is not hungry for breakfast, it may be that he is eating his bedtime snack too late or in too much volume. Keep the snack small (i.e. ½ portions of protein and carbohydrates) and aim for having them 30-60 minutes before bedtime.

C - Clean Water: Notice the different ways friends and family members get their water intake; some may drink tap water, some may buy bottled and some may have a filter.

E - Eat for Health: Though working to help your child shed excess body fat, it is important that you supply sufficient amounts of healthy fat. Protein Types need a small amount of fat (i.e. olive oil, coconut oil, butter, the fats from nuts and seeds, avocado) at each meal or snack while other body types also need those types of fats but in smaller amounts.

Day-at-a-Glance Guidelines
Find Your BALANCE—Day 7

> **TIP of the day:**
>
> *Tomorrow you begin a mild dietary cleanse. You will need positive effort—remember KIB has never promised there would be no work, only that the work would be simple—but it will be well worth it.*

What's On the Menu?

Food Formula: today is the last day of eating small amounts of grains, sugars and fruit.

Managing the Day

B - Body Type: Family members may have varied body types but everyone can benefit from days 8-21 of **Find Your BALANCE**. Keep a variety of vegetables in the house for everyone, as well as the heavier proteins (red meats and healthy cheeses) that Protein Types do well on and the vegetable proteins (nuts, seeds and legumes) that Carbohydrate Types need.

A - Attitude: Though the goals and motivators children choose are generally shorter than longer term, today is a good day to look at some of the long term benefits of **Find Your BALANCE** and making *KIB* principles part of your life forever. Talk about the importance of being a healthy, active adult and being able to tackle activities such as keeping up with your child at the park.

L - Laughter/Play: Even in a busy day, make room for down time. Grab time after supper or when your child comes home from school to chat and catch up with each other's day.

A - Activity: If your child has any type of physical challenge that impacts her ability to be as physically active as others, do the best you can. The *KIB* program works well with children even if initially, the excess weight makes it difficult for a child to exercise (i.e. child uses a wheel chair and excess weight prohibits one parent alone being able to take her swimming). As weight decreases, it is often easier to help your child with physical activity.

N - Night's Sleep: If your child has previously had trouble sleeping, see if there have been any changes this past week as she has begun transitioning to a healthier style of eating.

C - Clean Water: When your child comes in from outdoor activity and wants a snack, start with a glass of water. It will re-hydrate her after the exercise and help her determine whether or not she is truly hungry or was simply thirsty.

E - Eat for Health: Ensure menu plans and shopping lists for days 8-21 of **Find Your BALANCE** are completed and that ingredients are ready to go for the start of *KIB*'s exciting next phase!

Day-at-a-Glance Guidelines
Find Your BALANCE—Day 8

> **TIP of the day:**
>
> *Decorate the table for supper tonight. It adds to the positive energy and makes everyone feel that much more celebratory. KIB wants you to enjoy the journey to health!*

Managing the Day

B - Body Type: Even though you likely have more than one body type represented in your home, everyone can benefit from a sugar/refined grain cleanse. However, be aware that different body types will experience different challenges. Protein Body Types may find the initial transition more challenging but often settle into the cleanse more quickly than the Mixed or Carbohydrate Body Types, who generally function best with at least a small amount of grains and/or starchy vegetables in their regular diet. Be supportive and acknowledge each individual's experience.

A - Attitude: As a loving parent, you may worry you are asking too much of your child for the next two weeks. While it is a challenge, I have seen family after family succeed at the last 2 weeks of **Find Your BALANCE** with amazing results. Children who make it all the way through **Find Your BALANCE** are so proud of having achieved this goal—they stand taller, feel more in control and are supercharged for the journey ahead.

L - Laughter/Play: Make sure to give your child time to decompress today—play a favourite card or board game with him and look for ways to get your child laughing. Whatever you do, make sure to have eye contact with your child and let him see that you believe in him!

A - Activity: While the *KIB* approach is to hold off on significantly increasing physical activity until some weight loss has occurred, activity can be a wonderful distraction during cleanse. Go for a family walk or visit the local pool.

N - Night's Sleep: This week, you will observe any changes in your child's sleep pattern. Make sure to have your child record hours of sleep in a daytimer or on the *How Am I Doing? Chart* (p. 221 or download from www.kidsinbalance.net/kib-resources-1.html).

C - Clean Water: Water is now your child's number one drink. Make sure he has his water bottle when he heads out today.

E - Eat for Health: Your menu plan for the last two weeks of **Find Your BALANCE** should include many foods and flavours familiar to your family. If you are adding new recipes, make sure they are ones most likely to be a hit with your child.

Day-at-a-Glance Guidelines
Find Your BALANCE—Day 9

TIP of the day:

If you do not already have some, buy colourful and convenient containers (see p. 56 for non-chemical leaching numbers) to use for packing lunches. Let your child pick her favourite colours!

Managing the Day

B - Body Type: Observe the responses and experiences of the different body types in your family. Is one grumpier than the other? Is one more energetic? These responses can be indicators of people's relationship to the fuel they require (i.e. getting used to less widely fluctuating blood sugar levels).

A - Attitude: This is as much a mental and emotional journey as it is a physical one. We tend to develop emotional connections to and mental reliance on the foods we eat. Food may provide comfort, companionship, pleasure or encouragement. When we remove some items, we feel as though we have lost those emotional and mental payoffs. If this is your child's experience, be ready to help her find other sources to draw on emotionally.

L - Laughter/Play: Remember that spontaneity is good and that play does not have to be anything planned. Just be ready to laugh or ham it up with your child when a moment presents itself.

A - Activity: When it has been a long day, the additional stress of this lifestyle change can feel overwhelming. If you are sensing low spirits, encourage your child to do something she really loves to do (i.e. walk to a friend's place), even if it is very sedentary (i.e. curl up with a favourite movie). This is a big transition and there is plenty of time ahead to get moving more vigorously.

N - Night's Sleep: Maintain regular and healthy sleep patterns, especially during this transition. Help your child ease into bedtime by allowing time to decompress, particularly in the hour or two before she goes to sleep. Depending upon your child's age, a favourite book, a cuddle with a parent, a board game or some colouring can all help her to quiet down and relax for the night.

C - Clean Water: Do not be afraid to give your child gold stars for every glass of water she consumes. Rewards for reaching certain milestones can be very helpful motivators.

E - Eat for Health: For the second week of **Find Your BALANCE**, if you are concerned your child will be hungry, pack a couple extra protein and veggie snacks. Your child may need them on occasion but generally she will realize this new way of eating keeps her satisfied until the next snack time or mealtime.

Day-at-a-Glance Guidelines
Find Your BALANCE—Day 10

> **TIP of the day:**
>
> *Kids often enjoy using kitchen gadgets, so pick up a couple of new, interesting ones. Whether it is a funky lemon juicer or a razzmatazz vegetable chopper, it can help make meal prep more fun for all.*

Managing the Day

B - Body Type: Different body types can exhibit different reactions throughout a cleanse. Look for symptoms such as bloating, lack of mental clarity, fatigue, lethargy, moodiness or blues as signs that toxins are making their way out of the body. Additional symptoms may include skin rashes, headaches, nausea, and changes in bowel movements. Symptoms should subside before the end of the first week. If not, review **Find Your BALANCE** FAQs (p. 89) on minimizing cleanse symptoms and/or contact your healthcare practitioner as symptoms may be unrelated to cleanse.

A - Attitude: If your child says it is too hard, do not be afraid to wholeheartedly agree with the fact that the last two weeks of **Find Your BALANCE** can be challenging. Just be quick to declare that you do not believe it is too hard for your child. Tell him how amazed you are with what he has already accomplished over the past couple of days and encourage him to stick it out for three more days, and see how he feels then. Speak the words, "You can do this. You **are** doing this!"

L - Laughter/Play: Celebrate at dinner tonight—three days into the last part of **Find Your BALANCE** is a milestone. Play a rousing game of "Simon Says" right at the dinner table.

A - Activity: Weather permitting, take an after-dinner family walk, even if it is only for 20 minutes. With younger kids, turn it into a game of Follow the Leader. It is a fun and painless way to get physical movement happening.

N - Night's Sleep: Medical studies find connections between sleep deprivation and weight gain; primarily, people who sleep less tend to show a higher percentage of weight gain. Make it a priority to get your child to bed on time.

C - Clean Water: Make sure your child is taking a water bottle to school today. Avoiding plastics? Check out stainless steel options (i.e. www.kleankanteen.com or www.nathansports.com).

E - Eat for Health: Make sure you are using fragrant ingredients to enhance the mealtime experience. Buy fresh instead of dried herbs. Have your child squeeze the lemon for a dressing recipe. Interaction with colourful, aromatic foods will make the eating experience all the more enjoyable.

Day-at-a-Glance Guidelines
Find Your BALANCE—Day 11

> **TIP of the day:**
>
> *Have you remembered to pack an encouraging note in your child's lunch? Tell her how proud you are of her or simply create a silly limerick or poem.*

Managing the Day

B - Body Type: Any Protein Type family members may already be experiencing positive change—reduced sugar cravings and, increased energy—or they may simply be easily relaxing into this new routine. These are all signs that the cleansing benefits of **Find Your BALANCE** are taking effect.

A - Attitude: Despite these positive changes, your child may have trouble with the concept that this cleanse goes on for more than a few days. If she is struggling, invite her to help you plan a special celebration for Day 7. You could go to the pool, see a favourite movie or just party—cleanse-friendly style, of course. This will help shift her focus ahead to a goal.

L - Laughter/Play: Get your child to look up a few funny video clips on YouTube and have the whole family watch them together.

A - Activity: Household chores provide fantastic functional fitness, complete with stretching, lifting, twisting and running. Have plans to get your child involved in tasks around the house—it is good for her health and contributes to your child's future as a capable adult.

N - Night's Sleep: The old adage is still true: "Early to bed, early to rise, makes a man healthy, wealthy and wise." In bed before 11 p.m. and up before 7 a.m. are great guidelines. For children, depending upon age, back up the bedtime to 8, 9 or 10 p.m.

C - Clean Water: Water supports many important functions inside our bodies. It promotes the delivery of oxygen to our cells, contributes to the strength of our immune system and helps us digest and get rid of body waste! These are all powerful reasons to drink appropriate amounts of water on a daily basis.

E - Eat for Health: You are definitely spending more time in the kitchen and that can take some getting used to. Healthy food generally means it has not been pre-processed, pre-packaged or prepared by a manufacturer, which means more work for you. You will find as this week goes on, however, that it is not as much work as you may have originally thought. Also, you can find some peace in the fact that you are deliberately taking time each day to focus on your family's health. Keep up the good work!

Day-at-a-Glance Guidelines
Find Your BALANCE—Day 12

TIP of the day:

When time is in short supply, consider keeping a huge tightly sealed container of bite-sized vegetables on hand, so your child can quickly grab a snack on the run.

Managing the Day

B - Body Type: Do not underestimate the emotional dependency your child has on refined sugars and grains. You may see signs that indicate withdrawal from this highly addictive compound. Even once the physical cravings reduce, the emotional gap left by these foods may still challenge your child. Offer healthy solutions (i.e. parent time).

A - Attitude: How are you doing? Are you able to maintain a positive attitude and stay on top of **Find Your BALANCE** tasks? If you need support, review *KIB* material or FAQs. Your health—physical, emotional and spiritual—sets the tone for the rest of your family. *KIB* resources are designed to inspire a positive and encouraging tone.

L - Laughter/Play: A great game to get everyone talking around the dinner table is "Best and Worst." Each family member takes a turn sharing the best thing and the worst thing they experienced that day. It sparks laughter and provides opportunity for great support.

A - Activity: A fabulous foul weather activity is rebounding. Remember those mini-trampolines that were all the rage in the 80s? They're back and better than ever. Hundreds of muscles are worked while you jump and you can easily bounce while watching one of your favourite shows.

N - Night's Sleep: If your child has sleep challenges, you may want to take stock of the amount of active electronics in your child's room. A computer, a charging cell phone and a plugged-in alarm clock all send out electronic waves (EMFs) which research suggests may disrupt sleep patterns. Clear out the electronics and see whether it makes a difference.

C - Clean Water: Sometimes dehydration can masquerade as hunger. If your child is complaining of hunger, and he has recently had a snack or meal, encourage him to first drink a glass of water. Wait for 10 minutes. Often, the hunger pains disappear as the body's true need is met.

E - Eat for Health: Vegetables can be the hardest foods to keep interesting. In fact, you have likely gone through your list of options many times over by now. Do not worry; not only will you find new recipes over time but your family's taste buds will continue to expand to include vegetables previously not on the list of favourites.

Day-at-a-Glance Guidelines
Find Your BALANCE—Day 13

Managing the Day

B - Body Type: We cannot determine when and how quickly the body attends to specific issues. *KIB* kids have taken 10 months to lose 15 pounds; others shed double that in 3 months. Accept that a body will move at a pace of its choosing—simply take actions toward health on a consistent, daily basis.

A - Attitude: Keep examining whether any challenges are emotional—sadness at diminished food choices—or physical—fewer sugar highs. Understanding can lead to better food/activity choices.

L - Laughter/Play: At dinner, ask each family member to describe a moment in their day when they laughed. If someone hasn't yet had a chuckle, see if others can help!

A - Activity: Moving a little every day during cleanse helps the body release toxins. Make sure to work in even a 15-20 minute family walk.

N - Night's Sleep: A European study[1] on teen cell phone use compared light cell phone users—fewer than 5 calls/texts per day—with heavy users—more than 15 calls/texts per day. Heavy users:

- Had a harder time getting up in the morning. They woke at 10:50 a.m., on average, vs. 8:34 a.m. for the light users.
- Woke up more often during the night.
- Spent more time tossing and turning before falling asleep.
- Drank more soft drinks that pack a punch of caffeine and drank more alcohol.

C - Clean Water: Did you know water helps regulate body temperature?

E - Eat for Health: Protein-rich foods come in many forms and though some children are reluctant to embrace legumes, they are a wonderful, fibre-filled protein option that is a good source of B-complex vitamins, iron, potassium and zinc. Their nutritional balance of carbohydrates and protein means they do not cause a spike in blood sugar and they give a satisfying full feeling, which is great for Protein Body Types. Hummus anyone?

Day-at-a-Glance Guidelines
Find Your BALANCE—Day 14

> **TIP of the day:**
>
> *To make a meal special, visit the dollar store to find decorations for a celebratory themed dinner. You can go with the standard Mexican or Luau theme, or you can get creative, grab a permanent marker and turn "Graduate!" balloons into "Find Your BALANCE Graduate!"*

Managing the Day

B - Body Type: After one week, physical changes could be evident, and not simply weight loss alone. Look first for evidence of improved focus, clear mind, upbeat mindset, increased energy, less bloating and a feeling of overall lightness and well being.

A - Attitude: Time to present your child's weekly motivator. Do so with flourish and articulate what he has achieved or a particular choice that really impressed you.

L - Laughter/Play: This is a great night to pull out a favourite family board game. A crazy game of Cranium or Apples to Apples is a great way to be silly and celebrate.

A - Activity: Look for seasonal fun—a snow fort if it is winter, badminton in the summer.

N - Night's Sleep: It is easy for life to get hectic; some nights it seems as though everyone is busy right up until the clock strikes bedtime. Be committed to clearing time for your child to decompress before bedtime; do your best to stick to a healthy bedtime routine.

C - Clean Water: Water is an amazing thing. It often seems that the more you drink an appropriate amount, the more your body craves. Keep at it!

E - Eat for Health: Some parents feel their child eats enough vegetables, even if he is only eating lots of cucumber. That is a great start, but a variety of vegetables—including dark leafy greens—are required to provide balanced nutrients for the body.

1 c./100g serving	Calcium	Vit A	Vit C	Iron	Beta C	Folate	Fibre	Calories
Cucumber	n/a		6mg	n/a	trace	trace	n/a	15
Broccoli	75 mg		100%RDA	1.2 mg		20%RDA	3.5 g	44
Carrots		100%RDA			18 mg		4 g	70

Because of their high water content, cucumbers are low in calories, but do not miss out on the calcium and Vitamin C from broccoli, and the beta-carotene and Vitamin A from carrots. Keep mixing it up, giving variety and following the "one taste" guideline.

> **TIP of the day:**
>
> *The Dove Campaign has an amazing website that covers issues such as girls' body esteem and self-acceptance. They even have a workbook for mothers and daughters to use to more effectively dialogue about this topic. Visit www.campaignforrealbeauty.com.*

Managing the Day

B - Body Type: Help your child find the good things about her body. She may be carrying extra weight but she is likely sturdy and strong. A larger size can be a good thing! Often Protein Body Types have beautiful skin and are challenged with fewer blemishes than other body types. Does your child have thick hair, or is she flexible? From eyesight to hearing to the ability to reach the top shelf without a chair, we all have lots for which to be thankful.

A - Attitude: There are many things in life we cannot control. The Prayer of St. Francis of Assisi still resonates today—we find peace in accepting the things we cannot change and courageously face the things we can. Help your child focus on the things that are within her circle of control and set small but achievable goals for change. As change happens, goals can grow; that reality is a powerful motivator for your child to take into adult life.

L - Laughter/Play: Put out an assortment of vegetables and protein-rich foods in all shapes and sizes, and encourage your child and her friends to create veggie art. Award each one a prize (i.e. most colourful). The catch—they need to use reasonable proportions and eat what they make!

A - Activity: Yard work is fantastic functional fitness and a breath of fresh air is usually revitalizing. If seasonally applicable, enlist all family members in an outdoor clean up. Live in a townhouse or apartment? Volunteer to help out in a friend or neighbour's yard.

N - Night's Sleep: As we age, adults can have increasing difficulty with sleep-maintenance insomnia (i.e. staying asleep all night). Limit caffeine and alcohol, and keep the bedroom for relaxing activities only (i.e. do not do work or watch the news in bed).

C - Clean Water: If your child is craving juice or pop, make lemonade with water, freshly squeezed lemon juice and stevia to taste. In warmer weather, you could even add crushed ice and a splash of club soda to create your own slushie.

E - Eat for Health: Lunches taste so much better when they are well packed. Have a good-sized ice pack to keep things cold and use tightly sealed containers for added freshness.

Day-at-a-Glance Guidelines
Find Your BALANCE—Day 16

TIP of the day:

If motivation is lagging, surprise your child with a cleanse-friendly treat in his lunch. A tasty new veggie dip or a small spontaneous serving of Maple Ricotta Pudding (p. 178) can brighten a day.

Managing the Day

B - Body Type: If you have not done so for a few days, run through *KIB's Food/Mood/Activity Log* with your child to assess how he is feeling. Compare results with a *Food/Mood/Activity Log* completed prior to week three of **Find Your BALANCE**. You should see noticeable change.

A - Attitude: It is easy to be disappointed when a family member does not follow **Find Your BALANCE** exactly as it is laid out. Rather than focusing on the negative, however, keep an ongoing list of each person's successes. Spontaneously point out these successes, letting family members know how impressed you are with their choices; encourage more of them.

L - Laughter/Play: *America's Got Talent* (or not!) is a wonderful way to get the whole family laughing. Record it and watch the show later, at a time that works for everyone.

A - Activity: Walking stairs is a wonderful source of exercise—the activity not only elevates heart rate but also helps build important muscles in the body. If you have a sturdy set of stairs in your house, encourage your child to walk up and down them for a certain amount of time. Start with perhaps 5 minutes and work up to 10 minutes, having your child record how many flights he walked or ran in that time period.

N - Night's Sleep: Is your child a hot sleeper (i.e. does he often wake up with the sheets damp from sweat)? If so, a sheepskin mattress cover is a great solution. It allows air to circulate under and around the body and is a worthwhile, long-lasting investment.

C - Clean Water: Are you still tracking your child's water consumption?

E - Eat for Health: Some people are afraid that pursuing a healthy lifestyle means giving up red meat. Not so! Red meat is a protein-rich super food and a major source of micronutrients, including iron, vitamin B12, niacin and zinc. Red meat contains saturated fats, but provided animals have been grass-fed and raised naturally, without medication, the saturated fat content and essential fatty acid ratio suit most Mixed Body Types and usually all Protein Body Types. Carbohydrate Body Types should limit the quantity and frequency of their red meat intake and instead more often consume lighter and leaner protein sources such as chicken breast, light fish and legumes.

TIP of the day:

A favourite KIB kitchen gadget is the hand blender. It is wonderful for blending soups or whisking eggs to a quick froth. The chopper attachment is perfect for dicing ingredients for sauces or dressings, making food preparation quick and (almost) painless!

Managing the Day

B - Body Type: Protein Body Types often show early **Find Your BALANCE** change with a slightly slimmed down face. Energy levels and mood may also be more upbeat than before the cleanse. Hold off on taking any measurements until **Phase 1 – Find Your BALANCE** is over.

A - Attitude: When a positive attitude is not readily available, we create the possibility for it by the words we choose. Be alert for ways you can re-frame potentially negative situations. If your child tells you that they hate **Find Your BALANCE**, first sincerely acknowledge the emotion. Then respond with something like, "To hear you say you hate this phase and to know that you have stuck with it, makes me so proud of you! How do you do it?"

L - Laughter/Play: As busy parents, we often miss opportunities presented by our children to laugh or play. Whether it is a story about their day or a 15-minute break to challenge each other at Wii tennis, when chance for a "play date" happens, do not miss out.

A - Activity: Walking instead of driving is a positive choice for both our physical health and our environment. Think about places you could walk where you would normally drive and take advantage of an easy way to get your 30 minutes of activity for the day.

N - Night's Sleep: Pillows can make a huge difference between a restful and a restless sleep. If your child is having trouble sleeping, try experimenting with different pillows. There are many options available (i.e. feather, wool, synthetics). Talk to an expert for advice.

C - Clean Water: Start the day with water. The benefits are huge: it can help flush toxins the body has been processing throughout the night and support your kidneys' many healthful actions.

E - Eat for Health: Calorie counting—a less-than-natural, and potentially harmful, way of handling childhood obesity—is not *KIB*'s first line of defence. Unless portions are inappropriately large, if your child eats a proper fuel mix of nutrient dense and fibrous foods until comfortably full, and is active, she should lose fat. Only if good choices are being made and a fat loss plateau occurs for more than 3-4 weeks would a more careful evaluation of energy (i.e. caloric) intake and expenditure seem prudent. Even then, with children it is usually best to increase activity, not decrease food.

Day-at-a-Glance Guidelines
Find Your BALANCE—Day 18

Managing the Day

B - Body Type: No matter body type, everyone is negatively affected by eating refined sugar. It contains empty calories and no fibre, minerals or proteins. This forces your body to borrow vital nutrients—calcium, potassium and magnesium—from healthy cells elsewhere in your body to metabolize the sugar. Over time, as more and more nutrients are required to correct the imbalance, depletion occurs. Refined sugars are an equal-opportunity health destroyer. Encourage your Carbohydrate and Mixed Types to stick to **Find Your BALANCE** as firmly as your Protein Types.

A - Attitude: Speak out the truth of what you are doing for yourselves as a family. Congratulate each other for making health a priority and for coming this far!

L - Laughter/Play: Have a joke-off. Everyone brings a joke to share at the dinner table. Vote to see whose joke was the funniest, but remember, you cannot vote for your own.

A - Activity: Did you know that having more lean tissue and muscle in your body means your body will burn more energy, even while sleeping? The increase in burning ability is not huge and it will need to offset the fact your child is carrying less weight and therefore will have a lower Resting Metabolic Rate (p. 101), but every bit counts. Finding ways to build muscle strength in your child is a powerful way to move him forward.

N - Night's Sleep: Sleep is especially important for teenagers, who should get an average of 9 hours per night in the summer months and about 9.5 hours in winter. Growth hormones, crucial to their development throughout puberty, are secreted during sleep.

C - Clean Water: If your child broke a sweat today, he needs to compensate with additional water. Mild dehydration can produce symptoms such as dizziness, fatigue and a slight headache over the eyes. Young children are particularly susceptible to dehydration and should be taught that water, rather than sugar and chemical-laden sports drinks, is the best drink to replenish their bodies.

E - Eat for Health: Plan the menu for Day 21. It is a good opportunity to review items that have been hits and items that can be dropped. Alternatively, you can pull out the cookbooks or search the Internet to find a tantalizing new cleanse-friendly recipe.

Day-at-a-Glance Guidelines
Find Your BALANCE—Day 19

> **TIP of the day:**
>
> *Surprisingly, protein is often the food item least represented at a social gathering or a friend's house. Starches and perhaps vegetable trays are more usual snacks of choice. Having a few pepperoni sticks, some cleanse-friendly Trail Mix (p. 123) or cheese strings in tow, helps your child feel in control.*

Managing the Day

B - Body Type: If you have not yet begun to do so, it is time to start planning ahead for next week's menu. Now that you know the different Body Types represented in your family, you will want to review *KIB*'s information on *Fuel Mix Guidelines* (p. 187) so you can prepare for individual needs.

A - Attitude: If there is an event where your child will have to say no to a much-loved treat, remind her that it is only for the present. In the future, when your family is in balance, she will know how to create a place for Sometimes Foods while at the same time never giving up the health she has so diligently earned.

L - Laughter/Play: Playing friendly pranks on each other is a wonderful way to create positive energy. Find a way to surprise your family with a gag—setting alarm clocks a ½ hour early, leaping out of the laundry hamper when someone least expects it or . . . ?

A - Activity: Only a few days left to go. If you need a distraction or want to flush toxins out of your system, go for a family bike ride or take your child hiking or ice-skating.

N - Night's Sleep: REM sleep is said to activate the part of the brain connected with learning. While you sleep, the brain encodes recently acquired information and stores it for future use. That is why all-nighters before exams never really work that well!

C - Clean Water: Mom was right: drinking 6-11 glasses [1.5 litres-2.75 litres] of water a day is a great idea. What she might not have told you, however, is that while the amount of water intake is important, the quality of the water is also important. Start with tap water, but as opportunity avails, switch to filtered or bottled water. With the latter, use glass or at the least, avoid plastics numbered 2, 4, 5 and non-polycarbonate 7.

E - Eat for Health: Studies indicate that mindless TV watching can produce mindless eating. With rare exception (i.e. Olympics), keep the TV off during mealtimes and limit screen time in general.

Day-at-a-Glance Guidelines
Find Your BALANCE—Day 20

TIP of the day:

On a day when you have the time, pre-make all the items you needs for a portable supper. You, the food preparer, will actually feel like you get the evening off by completely removing yourself from the kitchen. A change really is as good as a rest!

Managing the Day

B - Body Type: Make sure the different body types in your family know what to expect as they enter **Build Your BALANCE**. Hopefully, you have reinforced throughout *KIB*'s first phase that life after a cleanse of this type does not go back to what it was before **Find Your BALANCE**; this is a change that moves you forward to a new way of doing life. Having said that, your child will enjoy choosing where in the day he will place his grain or starchy vegetable and fruit serving(s).

A - Attitude: Do up certificates of achievement on the computer or by hand for your family members. Everyone can suggest a particular achievement they observed in family members and you can take turns presenting them at tomorrow night's celebration.

L - Laughter/Play: Sometimes changing your usual eating locale can revitalize everyone. If the weather permits, why not pack a picnic to take to the local park. Meat kabobs, a yummy salad and a vegetable platter suddenly seem much more fun. If it is too cold outside, clear space in the family room and have your child set up a picnic on the floor.

A - Activity: A picnic supper in the park is a wonderful excuse to be active before and after your meal. Bring along a Frisbee or football and have some good old-fashioned fun playing catch.

N - Night's Sleep: After an evening outside, even if it is only for an hour, everyone seems to sleep a little better. There is nothing like fresh air to get you ready for a good night's sleep.

C - Clean Water: A big jug of water with ice and lemon is easy to take along on your picnic. You might even pack a few pre-filled water balloons for a creative alternative use for water.

E - Eat for Health: The great thing about **Find Your BALANCE** suppers is that they are quite conducive to eating outdoors. Bunless burgers, pre-cooked and chilled pork tenderloin or even tuna salad can all make wonderful main stage appearances for a portable meal. Be creative, and think outside the dining room!

TIP of the day:

While celebrating today, make sure to clarify for your family that life does not go back to the way it was before **Find Your BALANCE**. *You are all moving forward into a new way of living and caring for your bodies—a new "normal"! Make sure everyone knows what is coming in the weeks ahead.*

Managing the Day

B - Body Type: With measurements coming up tomorrow, this is a good time to remind your child that every body responds differently to lifestyle change. While one body may lose lots of weight during cleanse, another may not lose a pound but will instead have lost an inch [2 cm] around the abdominal area. Another may have found health benefits such as better moods or more energy. Either way, every body profits from a break from refined sugars and grains and will gain even more benefit when moving ahead with predominately complex sources of carbohydrates (i.e. starchy vegetables, whole grains, vegetables) from this point on.

A - Attitude: Have some fun with the presentation of certificates of achievement, encouraging each family member to say a little something when making the presentation. Do not forget to give each other a big round of applause.

L - Laughter/Play: In addition to the certificates, you can play "Best and Worst" for **Find Your BALANCE**. That should bring up a few laughs (i.e. a recounting of when Mom tried to serve asparagus at breakfast or a sibling had to say "no thank you" fourteen times to Grandma's pleas to indulge in her world famous plum pudding).

A - Activity: Dancing is a fantastic way to get your heart rate up. Crank the tunes and shake it up. You will be practising a great combination of celebration and activity.

N - Night's Sleep: Everyone should hopefully sleep well tonight—**Find Your BALANCE** is over and a new phase begins.

C - Clean Water: With **Find Your BALANCE** ending, do not fall into the trap of incorporating juices, pop—either diet or regular—coffee or more than small amounts of milk into the dietary plan again. In **Build Your BALANCE** and beyond, the beverage of choice for your child—and indeed the whole family—should continue to be water.

E - Eat for Health: Ensure menu plans and shopping lists for **Build Your BALANCE** are completed and that ingredients and snacks are ready to go for the start of *KIB*'s next dietary phase!

Notes

The *KIB* Approach to Wellness

1. Sarah E. Anderson, PhD, Robert C. Whitaker, MD, MPH, "Household Routines and Obesity in US Preschool-Aged Children," *PEDIATRICS* Vol. 125 No. 3 March 2010, (doi:10.1542/peds.2009-0417): 420-428.
2. Nicola Kime, "Children's eating behaviours: the importance of the family setting," *Area* Vol. 40 No. 3, 2008: 315-322.
3. Diane Berry, Rebedda Sheehan, Rhonda Heschel, Kathleen Knafl, Gail Melkus, Margaret Grey, "Family-Based Interventions for Childhood Obesity: A Review," *Journal of Family Nursing* November 2004 vol. 10 no. 4: 429-449.

Seven Problems – Seven Solutions

1. Ebba Bråkenhielm, Renhai Cao, Bihu Gao, Bo Angelin, Barbara Cannon, Paolo Parini, Yihai Cao, "Angiogenesis Inhibitor, TNP-470, Prevents Diet-Induced and Genetic Obesity in Mice," *Circulation Research* 2004;94:1579.
2. HR Lijnen, "Angiogenesis and obesity," *Cardiovascular Research* 2008 May 1;78(2):286-293, Epub 2007 Aug 23.

Attitude

1. Kerry Kawakami, John F. Dovidio, Ap Dijksterhuis, "Effect of Social Category Priming on Personal Attitudes," *Psychological Science* Vol. 14, No. 4, July 2003.
2. Jennifer R. Steele, Nalini Ambady, ""Math is Hard!" The effect of gender priming on women's attitudes," *Journal of Experimental Social Psychology* 42 (2006): 428–436.
3. Larry Crabb, *The Marriage Builder*, Zondervan Publishing House, 1992: 74-75.

Laughter and Play

1. M. Buchowski, K. Majchrzak, K. Blomquist, K. Chen, D. Dyrne, J. Bachorowski, "Energy expenditure of genuine laughter," International Journal of Obesity (Lond), 2007 Jan;31(1):131-137, *Epub* 2006 May 2.
2. David S. Sobel, and Robert Ornstein, MD, *The Healthy Mind, Healthy Body Handbook*, NY: Patient Education Media, Inc., 1996: 49-59.
3. Research by William Fry Jr., PhD in Bruce Lipton, PhD. *The Biology of Belief*, CA: Mountain of Love/Elite Books, 2005: 197.
4. Mary O'Brien, MD, *Successful Aging*, CA:Biomed General, 2007: 152-153.

5. Lee S. Berk, Stanley A. Tan, Dottie Berk, "Cortisol and Catecholamines stress hormone decrease is associated with the behaviour of perceptual anticipation of mirthful laughter," *The FASEB Journal* 2008;22:946.11.

6. Lee S. Berk and Stanley A. Tan, "[beta]-Endorphin and HGH increase are associated with both the anticipation and experience of mirthful laughter," *The FASEB Journal* 2006;20:A382.

7. Charles C. Neuhoff, Charles Schaefer, "Effect of laughing, smiling, and howling on mood," *Psychological Reports* 202 Dec ;91 (3 Pt2):1079-1080.

Activity

1. J. Levine, "Non-exercise activity thermogenesis (NEAT)," *Best Practice & Research Clinical Endocrinology & Metabolism* 2002 Dec;16(4):679-702.

2. Al Sears, MD, *Rediscover Your Native Fitness, PACE,"* Wellness Research & Consulting, Inc., 2006.

3. Nielsen Three Screen Report; Q1 2010.

Sleep

1. *Tufts University Health & Nutrition Letter,* "You Snooze, You Lose?" April 2005: p. 6.

2. James E. Gangwisch, Dolores Malaspina, Bernadette Boden-Albala, Steven B. Heymsfield, "Inadequate Sleep as a Risk Factor for Obesity: Analyses of the NHANES I," *SLEEP*, Vol. 28, No. 10, 2005.

3. K. Spiegel, E. Tasali, P. Penev, E. Van Cauter, "Brief Communication: Sleep curtailment in healthy young men is associated with decreased leptin levels, elevated ghrelin levels, and increased hunger and appetite," *Annals of Internal Medicine* 2004;141:845-850.

4. S. Taheri, L. Lin, D. Austin, T. Young, E. Mignot, "Short sleep duration is associated with reduced leptin, elevated ghrelin, and increased body mass index," *PLoS Medicine* 2004;1:e62.

5. K. Spiegel, R. Leproult, E. Van Cauter, "Impact of sleep debt on metabolic and endocrine function," *Lancet* 1999;354:1435-1439.

6. Andy R. Ness, "The Avon Longitudinal Study of Parents and Children (ALSPAC) – a resource for the study of the environmental determinants of childhood obesity," *European Journal of Endocrinology* (2004) 151 U141–U149.

7. M. H. Repacholi, "WHO's International EMF Project," World Health Organization, Geneva, Switzerland, http://www.who.int/peh-emf/meetings/southkorea/en/M_H_Repacholi.pdf.

8. A.M. Adachi-Mejia, M.R. Longacre, J.J. Gibson, M.L. Beach, L.T Titus-Ernstoff, M.A. Dalton, "Children With a TV in Their Bedroom at Higher Risk for Being Overweight," *International Journal of Obesity* 2007; 31: 644–651.

9. Christelle Delmas, Carine Platat, Brigitte Schweitzer, Aline Wagner, Mohamed Oujaa and Chantal Simon, "Association Between Television in Bedroom and Adiposity Throughout Adolescence," *Obesity* (2007) **15**, 2495–2503; doi: 10.1038/oby.2007.296.

Clean Water

1. Brenda M. Davy, Elizabeth A. Dennis, Laura Dengo, Kelly L. Wilson and Kevin P. Davy, "Water Consumption Reduces Energy Intake at a Breakfast Meal in Obese Older Adults," *Journal of the American Dietetic Association* 2008 July; 108(7): 1236-1239; doi: 10.1016/j.jada.2008.04.013.

Eat for Health

1. Sharon P. Fowler, Ken Williams, Roy G. Resendez, Kelly J. Hunt, Helen P. Hazuda and Michael P. Stern, "Fueling the Obesity Epidemic? Artificially Sweetened Beverage Use and Long-term Weight Gain," *Obesity* (2008): 16 8, 1894-1900 doi:10.1038/oby.2008.284.
2. X. T. Wang and Robert D. Dvorak, "Sweet Future: Fluctuating Blood Glucose Levels Affect Future Discounting," *Psychological Science* February 2010 21:2: 183-188.
3. Frank Q. Nuttall and Mary C. Gannon, "Metabolic response of people with type 2 diabetes to a high protein diet," *Nutrition & Metabolism* (Lond) 2004: 1:6.
4. Heather Basciano, Lisa Federico and Khosrow Adeli, "Fructose, insulin resistance, and metabolic dyslipidemia," *Nutrition & Metabolism* 2005 2:5.

Worksheets

1. Thanks to Penny Ormsbee for her foundational work on *Kitchen Substitutes* and the *Healthy Food Lists*. Though the charts have been adapted from the originals for the *KIB* program, Penny's nutritional research and template set-ups saved me hours of work!
2. Michelle Hartte, *The Fit n Healthy Plan — The Nutritional Diet & Lifestyle Plan — Made Easy!*, ©Michelle Hartte, 2010. *Natural Sweetener* worksheet adapted from information in *The Fit n Healthy Plan* and used with permission.

Day-at-a-Glance Guidelines

1. Bader G, et al "Does excessive mobile phone use affect sleep in teenagers?" APSS Meeting 2008; Abstract 249, as cited in article by Michael Smith, "APSS: Heavy Cell Phone Use by Teens and Young Adults Linked to Poor Sleep," *MedPage Today* June 9, 2008.

Index
(Recipes are listed in **bold** type)

CPSIA information can be obtained at www.ICGtesting.com
Printed in the USA
236703LV00005B/11/P

9 780986 636509